need to know?

Running

D0434705

Alison Hamlett

Collins

First published in 2007 by Collins
an imprint of
HarperCollins Publishers
77–85 Fulham Palace Road
London W6 8JB

www.collins.co.uk

Collins is a registered trademark of HarperCollins Publishers Limited

11 10 09 08 07
6 5 4 3 2 1

A catalogue record for this book is available from the British Library

Editor: Heather Thomas
Designer: Rolando Ugolini
Series design: Mark Thomson
Photographs: Steven Seaton, Mike King, Nigel Farrow and Getty Images
Front cover photograph: Getty Images
Back cover photographs: Steven Seaton

ISBN-13: 978-0-00-723631-2
ISBN-10: 0-00-723631-X

Colour reproduction by Colourscan, Singapore
Printed and bound by Printing Express Ltd, Hong Kong

Contents

Introduction

Running is a very simple sport. It requires little, if any, special equipment. There are no courts to book or opponents to juggle your schedule around. You can do it almost anywhere, at any time and for as long or as little as you like. And, best of all, we all know how to do it – we don't need to learn how to run.

Benefits of running

However, despite its simplicity, running is also a powerful sport. It's the most effective form of exercise you can do, burning more calories per minute than any other form of aerobic activity. Regular runners also have a lower incidence of heart disease, certain kinds of cancers and lower stress levels than their sedentary counterparts. Running genuinely has the power to change lives and it can change yours, too.

New challenges

If you have never run before, this book will help you to take your first running steps. It will provide you with all the basic knowledge and inspiration that you need when you are starting out: from buying your first pair of running shoes to the best way to fit your running into a busy lifestyle. You will be surprised at how quickly you will improve. Today you might be out of breath walking up a flight of stairs but in just six short weeks – if you can commit 30 minutes three times a week to running – you could be taking part in your first race.

From there, the possibilities are endless – whether you want to challenge your competitive side or make running the active part of a healthier lifestyle. You will find information on all of these subjects and much more in the following pages. Learn everything from what you need to eat and drink to fuel your new hobby, to how to stay motivated so you never miss a run. This will add up to make you the best runner you can possibly be. Your new hobby will introduce you to physical and mental health benefits as well as new friends and opportunities. Welcome to a new you.

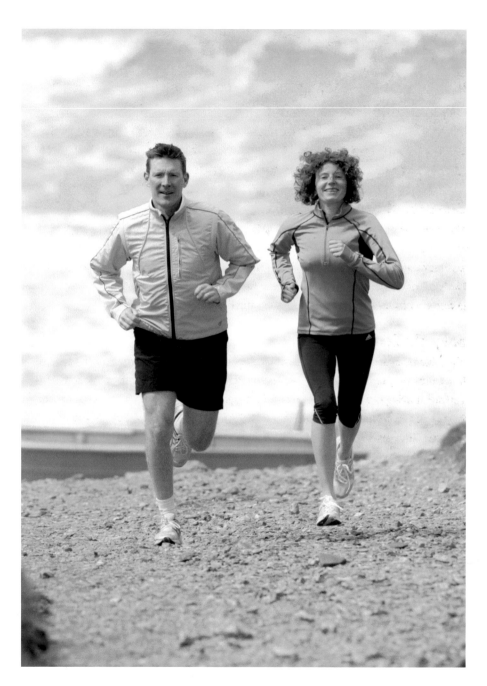

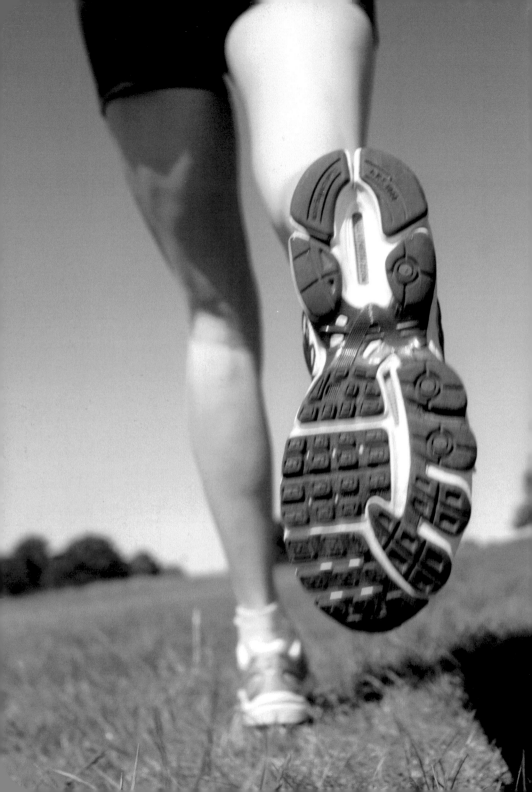

1 Getting started

Running is one of the simplest sports around. If you can walk, you can run, and all you really need to start out is a decent pair of running shoes and some enthusiasm. You can run any time and anywhere. Whatever the weather, you can enjoy a run alone or with friends. Once you start you will be surprised at how quickly your running improves. You will feel fitter, healthier, and full of energy and zest for life. Isn't it time you made running part of your life?

Make running part of your life

You've decided that you want to run – and that's great. In just a few short weeks you will be able to step out of your front door and run for more than half an hour. Before you get to that stage, however, you need to know how to make running part of your life.

must know

Plan ahead
If your diary becomes booked up days or even weeks in advance, schedule your runs just as you would any other meeting. By blocking out a chunk of time for your run, you'll get into the habit of approaching your training as non-negotiable.

Make it fun

Have you ever noticed how much fun children look as though they are having just running around? Try to inject some fun and originality into every run by doing something a little different. Run a favourite route in the opposite direction, set yourself a little goal, such as seeing how many other runners you can say hello to, or just sing to yourself. Lots of runners find that they enjoy a run much more if they have great music for company. A collection of your favourite tracks will put a spring in your step and take your attention away from the miles. Remember that you are more likely to stick with it when you are having a good time.

Get real

You may be so enthusiastic when you start running that you want to run every day, seven days a week. While it's great that you're so keen, you need to give your body time to adapt to your new routine or you might succumb to injury. Remember that running is a lifelong aim. Don't expect to be lining up at the start of the London Marathon with Paula Radcliffe on your next birthday – although that's possible, if it's really your goal. Take it slowly when you're starting out, and running will become a lifelong friend.

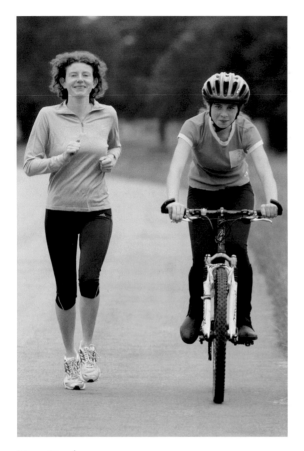

You will enjoy your new hobby even more if you involve your family and friends.

Don't give up

There will be times when you wonder why you are struggling through the rain or forcing yourself to run up a hill when the sofa looked so inviting, but don't give up. Anything worth doing is going to be tough, running included, but that's exactly what makes it all worthwhile in the end. Prepare to feel exhausted, frustrated and impatient, but use these emotions to motivate yourself. You always feel better after a run, and you will have more energy and a fresh perspective on life. Try it and find out for yourself.

Club together

Surround yourself with people who are passionate about running. You will be more likely to enjoy your new hobby and stick with it if you have enthusiastic friends to run with. Ask your family to support you, but, better still, find some training partners to share the miles. You will motivate each other to keep going and it will be more fun if you have a friend to talk to while you are out running.

Strike a balance

It will be easier to stick to your new routine if it fits in with the rest of your life. If you're constantly busy, finding time to run can be a struggle but with a little creativity you can make time. Drop your children at football practice and run around the pitch while they train. Try running to or from work once a week. Squeeze a 30-minute run into your lunch hour. Even getting up half an hour earlier than usual will give you time to run.

Close to home

Since you can run anywhere, make life easier by finding a place to run that's convenient. It does not matter a jot whether you run on a treadmill at the gym near work or explore the options close to your home: what matters is that you are out there doing it and making running part of your life.

Listen to your body

When you start to run it's natural that you will experience a few aches and pains as your body gradually adjusts to its new healthy regime. When this happens, just take a day off from running and

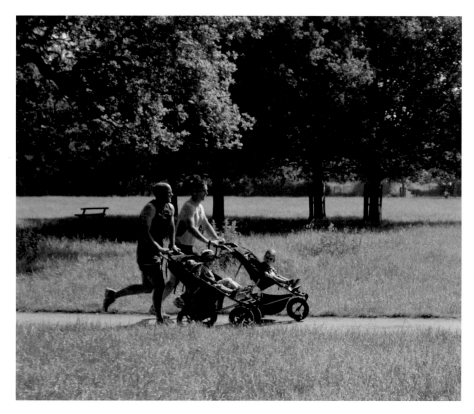

relax until your body has recovered. By giving it time to recuperate you are less likely to become injured and more likely to run regularly.

With a little creativity, it is easy to find time to run.

The danger zone

One of the most dangerous times in any runner's career is right at the beginning. You will improve rapidly, feel more fit and healthy, and be keen to enhance your experience by running faster and for longer. However, instead of running every day – which exposes you to potential injury and tiredness – try some different sports on days on which you're not scheduled to run.

Choosing the right shoes

Shoes are the one major purchase that every runner needs to worry about. Although sifting through the hundreds of pairs on offer might seem like a daunting prospect, you can narrow the choice with a little knowledge.

must know

What should I spend?
Running shoes can cost anywhere from £50 to £120, but cost is not the best indicator of a shoe's suitability for you. Your perfect shoes are the ones that fit properly, grip and protect your feet on all terrain and cause you no problems over a successful life together. Most runners find that mid-range shoes offer the best trade-off between value and technical sophistication.

Judging your foot type

Feet are like fingerprints – every set is unique. Nevertheless they fall into three main categories, and these are matched by three categories of running shoes. The classic method of judging your foot type is the wet test. Next time you step out of the shower look at the outline of your wet foot.
• A flat foot (a solid footprint with no discernible arch) usually means your foot rolls inwards after it hits the ground and needs the added support of a motion control shoe.
• A high-arched foot (the footprint has a narrow band connecting the front and the heel) generally doesn't roll inwards enough and needs a cushioned shoe which is also very flexible.
• A neutral foot (the footprint has a flare but shows the heel and forefoot firmly connected) should be matched with a stability shoe which has an equal blend of cushioning and stabilizing features. This is the most common category and applies to about 85 per cent of runners.

Shopping for shoes

Shopping at a specialist running retailer will make it far easier to determine your foot type and identify which shoes are best for you. These shops are staffed by runners who understand both the shoe market and the particular needs of beginners. They will measure and look at your feet, question you about the type of running you intend to do and will then recommend a selection of shoes for you to pick from.

Shop smart

Always shop in the afternoon when your feet have expanded to their largest size, and expect the process to take 20–30 minutes. Take along your old running shoes, if you have some – an experienced salesperson will be able to use them to assess what you need – as well as the socks you intend to run in. Try on both shoes and run around the shop in them, preferably for a few minutes. Don't rush the purchase or respond to sales pressure; you are the best judge of the right shoes for you.

When it comes to kit, your priority should be to buy a comfortable pair of running shoes that complement the way you run.

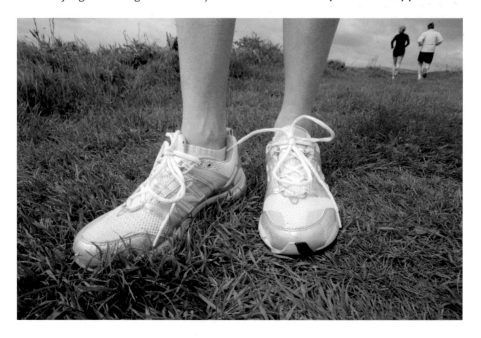

must know

Different surfaces
Stability, cushioned and motion control shoes are all designed for running and racing on roads and pavements. If you are going to do most of your running off-road, buy a trail shoe, which has a studded rubber outsole to give you better grip, and a tougher, more durable upper.

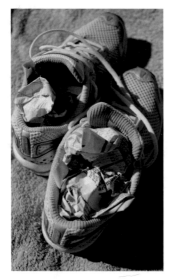

Stuff your shoes with newspaper to help them dry out.

Fit is everything

A shoe that doesn't fit you is the wrong shoe for you. A well-fitting running shoe will feel snug but not too tight, both in length and width. It should be sized to your bigger foot (if you have one) and have at least a thumbnail's worth of room between the end of your toes and the front of the shoe. The rear of the shoe should hold your heel firmly in place so that your foot does not slide around.

Treasure your shoes

Running shoes are designed for running, not for football, tennis or weight training. Although it might be tempting to use them for other sports, don't. Not only will you damage the structural integrity of your precious running shoes but you might also damage yourself as well. You can extend the life of your shoes with a little common sense when they are wet or dirty. When wet, put some scrunched-up newspaper inside and dry them slowly away from a direct heat source. When dirty, clean them with a brush and water, avoiding detergents, and never be tempted to put them in a washing machine.

Long life

There is no set lifespan for a pair of running shoes: it all depends on your weight, how your foot strikes the ground, whether you are running on or off roads, and also how well you care for the shoes themselves. Unlike your day shoes, the durability of running shoes is often dictated by the life of their midsole foam – not by the outsole rubber or the upper. Midsole wear can be very hard to judge, although heavy creasing of the foam under the heel, the feeling that your foot is sinking into the shoe or permanent flattening of the foam are all indicators that the time has come for some new shoes. You can reasonably expect your shoes to last between 300-500 miles, although some runners regularly manage twice as long.

Don't expect miracles

If you are expecting your shoes to make you a better and faster runner, you are deluding yourself. The shoes will not run the miles for you, but they can ensure that you run those miles comfortably and, hopefully, free of injury. Shoes that you never think about again until it's time to change them are the perfect ones for you.

must know

Try this
For a foolproof way of keeping your laces fastened during a run, try the fell runner's knot. Just tie the laces as though you were making a normal simple bow with a loop on either side of the middle. Before you pull the bow tight, take the right loop and feed it over and back on itself through the middle opening. Pulling on either loose lace will untie the bow.

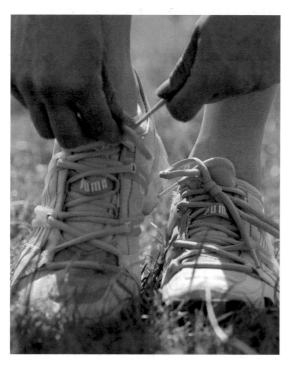

Your running shoes are the most important piece of kit you'll buy.

Understanding your shoe

The running shoe market is awash with technical terminology and jargon, but don't be confused by the scientific language; things are far more straightforward than you might imagine. To pinpoint the perfect shoe for you, you need to understand the basic features of a running shoe and the role each plays in helping you run injury free.

Insole
A removable liner inside the shoe, this helps with the fit and provides a little extra cushioning. Some runners with severe stability problems use a fitted, bespoke insole (orthoses) made by a podiatrist to correct the problem.

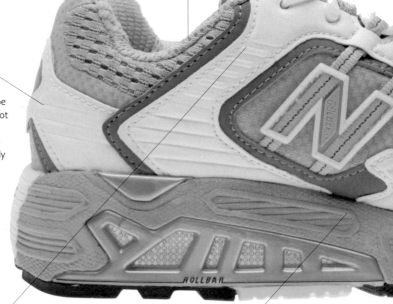

Heel counter
This is the firm area of material at the back of the shoe which keeps the foot firmly in place and stable. It should be rigid and sit vertically above the midsole.

Upper
This sits around and supports the foot; it should work with the midsole to control stability. If there is insufficient room in the front toebox, bruised black toenails are a common result.

Medial post
It should control any excessive foot movement and also provide shock absorption.

Laces

The primary role of the laces is to tie your foot into the upper. Different lacing systems can be used to customize the shoe to a wider or narrower foot or to relieve the pressure in certain areas. The tongue protects the foot from the pressure of the laces although you can find one-piece, slip-on uppers with fewer lace holes.

must know

Outsole

This rubber section of the shoe, which comes into contact with the ground and provides grip and traction, will rarely wear out before the midsole, although in time it will show signs of wear on the outer edge of the heel and on the forefoot.

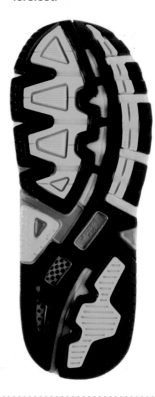

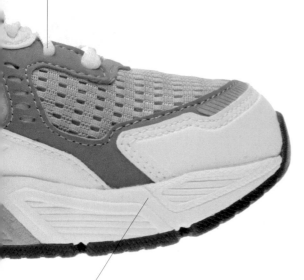

Midsole

The technical heart of the shoe made from foam (EVA or PU) that usually contains a company's trademark technical features, such as Nike's Air or Asics Gel. It should control excessive foot movement and provide shock absorption. Stability shoes have harder foams on the rear inside edge of the midsole; heavier motion control shoes also have extra support features.

Essential kit

Although you could run in any shorts and a cotton T-shirt, most people soon find that running is easier and more comfortable when they wear specifically designed running equipment.

must know

Sunglasses
These are increasingly important for runners. They protect eyes from damaging ultraviolet sunlight, cut down glare and, with the right coloured lenses, improve your visibility. Yellow lenses work best with low light conditions, blue or brown with strong sunlight. They are not an item to skimp on because poor sunglasses are worse than wearing none at all because they fool the eye into thinking it is protected, with the result that the pupil dilates more, letting in harmful UV light.

T-shirts

If you are used to running in cotton T-shirts, your first run in a modern synthetic shirt or singlet is almost a religious experience. They are lighter, more comfortable and, importantly, will stay dryer as they 'wick' sweat away from your body to the outside of the material where it can evaporate. They are most effective when they fit close to your body. The two drawbacks of synthetic shirts are the cost – they tend to be quite expensive – and smell (body odour can linger in them if they are not washed regularly).

Shorts

As with shirts, the cotton short is a dying breed. Traditional nylon running shorts have a built-in under-liner and a high cut around the top of the leg. The more modern versions have longer, baggier designs, although the tighter-fitting cycle-type short is almost as popular, particularly with women runners. All use synthetic fibres that dry quickly. The important thing is that they feel comfortable and do not restrict your movement.

Socks

In recent years, running socks have become almost as abundant as shoes. The key role of the sock is to protect your foot from blisters, either through a

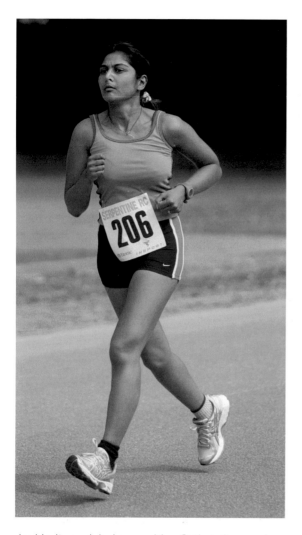

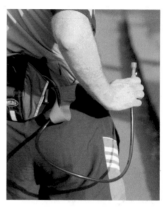

You can wear a vest and shorts in summer to keep you cool.

You can now choose from a vast range of accessories to make your running easier. This water carrier has its own drinking hose.

double-layered design or with a fit that sits snugly against your skin with no ridges and nowhere for the shoe to rub against your foot. Socks provide some extra cushioning under your heel or forefoot. In either case, opt for synthetic and wool mix materials that help move moisture away from your foot, so it stays dry and is less liable to blister.

must know

Water carriers
A hand-held bottle used to be the only way to carry water on a run, but now you can find dozens of specially designed belts, bottles and backpacks to make your life easier. Some even come with drinking hoses to make it yet simpler to take in fluid on the move.

Winter training gear

Good winter kit will make all-season running a pleasure rather than a chore. A good lightweight running jacket should be your main purchase. A breathable, windproof material that keeps you warm is more important than a completely waterproof layer that will not breathe as well. The fit should be close with enough space for an

Winter kit will help protect you from the elements when you are out running in cold weather.

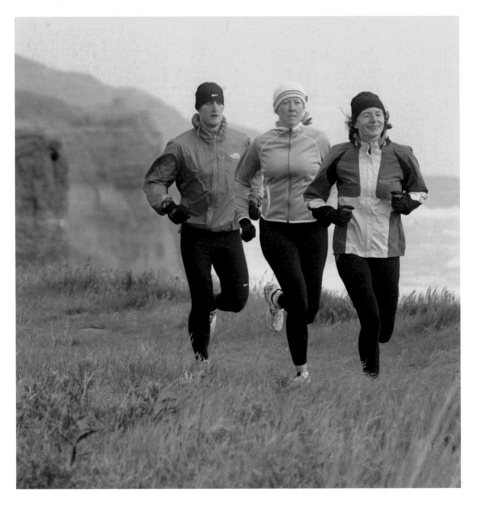

extra layer. Leggings are generally about warmth and comfort and come in tight or loose fittings.

Don't overdress for a winter run: you should feel a little cold at the start of the run because the running itself will warm you up. A sleeveless, windproof jacket (gilet) on top of a thermal base layer with leggings is enough for most people.

Layering

The secret of winter running is a good layering system. Start with a thin base layer that sits against your body and moves sweat from your skin to the outside of the material. The outer layer should be a thin shower-proof layer which also keeps the wind off. On particularly cold days, you can add a thermal fleece layer between the two. Several thin layers perform more efficiently than one thick one and will provide the flexibility you need to change your clothing with the weather conditions.

Women's kit

Technically, most women's kit is similar to that which is aimed at men; the chief differences are the fit and the designs. The single exception is the running sports bra – an item of equipment that is as important to any woman as her shoes. Sports bras come in a wide range of colours and sizes but generally will compress and support the breasts to limit movement. As with all sports equipment, the fit is key, but also look out for wide, non-slip straps, breathable material and a design that is comfortable to wear and does not restrict your movement.

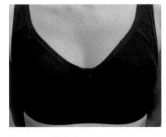

A supportive sports bra is an essential piece of kit for every female runner.

Running programmes

When you are starting out as a runner, do not make the mistake of thinking that walking is cheating. Every beginner's running programme starts with walking, and you will have to walk before you can run. Aim to begin by running for just 30 seconds, then walking until you have caught your breath, then repeating it.

must know

Run/walk
This is a great way for new runners to build up fitness, but it is a strategy that works for experienced runners, too. If you are coming back to running after an injury, run/walk is a great way to ease slowly back into training. Start running for one minute, then walking for one, and if everything feels fine, then increase the time you run without extending the walk break. Eventually you will be able to drop the walking entirely.

Walk to run

Even seasoned marathon runners throw a walk break into their running now and then, and with good reason. By alternating running with walking, you will give your body a chance to recover from the impact of running, because one of the main differences between running and walking is that in running you 'jump' off the ground. In walking, however, you don't, so there's much less impact on each foot strike and a reduced chance of injury.

Use your walk breaks to take in what's going on around you. Look at the view, enjoy the sun on your back or the rain on your face, and feel the ground beneath your feet.

Training benefits

When you start training using a run/walk schedule, not only will you help protect yourself from many common injuries, but you will also make greater improvements because you should be able to train for longer before you tire. If you can only run about 50 yards before becoming out of breath, you should walk for the next 50 yards to recover before starting to run again. Most first-timers who are new to the business of running start off by running too fast and too hard. It might last only a few minutes, but it's an experience that can put them off running forever. Walking is an easier and gentler introduction to running – it's more sustainable and will not leave you feeling disillusioned.

Talk test

Throughout your running training, you can also use the talk test to gauge whether you are going too fast. When you're starting out as a runner this is particularly useful. If you're too out of breath to chat to a training partner, slow down a little, and walk, until you get your breath back. Then start to jog but a little more slowly. This gentle approach will allow you to improve without denting your enthusiasm.

Mixing running with walking is a great way to stay motivated and improve rapidly.

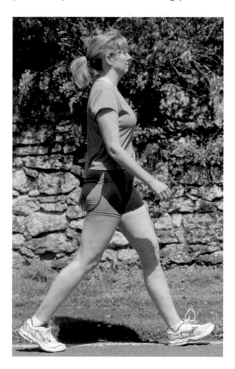
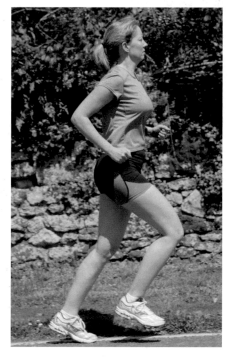

Beginner's programme

If you are completely new to running, the following programme will help you to run for 30 minutes in just six weeks. Stick to the schedule and you will be amazed at how quickly you improve.

Week 1

Monday:	Rest
Tuesday:	Run 30 seconds, walk 30 seconds. Repeat 20 times.
Wednesday:	Rest
Thursday:	Run 1 minute, walk 1 minute. Repeat 10 times.
Friday:	Rest
Saturday:	Rest
Sunday:	Run 2 minutes, walk 3 minutes. Repeat 5 times.

Week 2

Monday:	Rest
Tuesday:	Run 2 minutes, walk 2 minutes. Repeat 5 times.
Wednesday:	Rest
Thursday:	Run 3 minutes, walk 4 minutes. Repeat 4 times.
Friday:	Rest
Saturday:	Rest
Sunday:	Run 3 minutes, walk 3 minutes. Repeat 4 times.

Week 3

Monday:	Rest
Tuesday:	Run 4 minutes, walk 4 minutes. Repeat 4 times.
Wednesday:	Rest
Thursday:	Run 5 minutes, walk 5 minutes. Repeat 4 times.
Friday:	Rest
Saturday:	Rest
Sunday:	Run 5 minutes, walk 4 minutes. Repeat 4 times.

Week 4

Monday:	Rest
Tuesday:	Run 7 minutes, walk 4 minutes. Repeat 3 times.
Wednesday:	Rest
Thursday:	Run 7 minutes, walk 3 minutes. Repeat 3 times.
Friday:	Rest
Saturday:	Rest
Sunday:	Run 7 minutes, walk 2 minutes. Repeat 3 times.

Week 5

Monday:	Rest
Tuesday:	Run 9 minutes, walk 2 minutes. Repeat twice.
Wednesday:	Rest
Thursday:	Run 10 minutes, walk 2 minutes. Repeat twice.
Friday:	Rest
Saturday:	Rest
Sunday:	Run 12 minutes, walk 2 minutes. Repeat twice.

Week 6

Monday:	Rest
Tuesday:	Run 12 minutes, walk 2 minutes. Repeat twice.
Wednesday:	Rest
Thursday:	Run 15 minutes, walk 1 minute. Repeat twice.
Friday:	Rest
Saturday:	Rest
Sunday:	Run 30 minutes.

Getting ready to run

It's not enough to jump out of bed and pull your running shoes on: you need a little preparation before the start of every run. Follow these tips to ease effortlessly into the start of a run.

Warming up

You don't need to stretch before you run – in fact, research suggests that this might cause you more harm than good – but you do need to warm up the muscles that you are going to use. Start off with a brisk walk for five minutes before breaking into a gentle jog for another five minutes. You should start to feel warmer and ready to begin your training run.

If warming up outside in winter leaves you cold, you can cheat with a passive warm-up to increase the body's temperature without physical activity. Try a warm bath or heat packs, then run a little on the spot indoors before braving the outside world.

Cooling down

At the end of your run, do not stop until you have given your body a chance to cool down. Walking for five minutes after your run is an excellent way to deliver dynamic stretches to your muscles. You will find that it will reduce post-exercise stiffness more effectively than static stretching. Walk until you feel that your breathing has returned to normal.

Why stretch?

The jury is still out on whether stretching can offer any benefits for runners, but many people still like to stretch because they believe that it brings greater flexibility and makes them feel good. After a run your heart will be pumping blood and oxygen to your muscles, and a raised metabolic rate will speed up your nerve impulses, allowing for easier movement.

Getting going

One of the easiest mistakes to make when you are starting out as a runner is to run too fast. You remember what it was like to hare down the finishing straight on the athletics track at school and take off at a pace that you struggle to maintain for more than a couple of minutes. It's much easier to start slow and think about building up your speed when you can comfortably run for at least 30 minutes.

You should always save the stretching until after you have run – don't do it first.

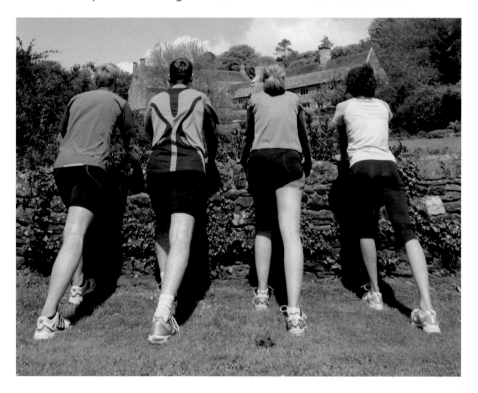

Stretching

You already know not to stretch before a run but if you want to stretch afterwards, walk until your heart rate and breathing have returned to normal, then stretch. Some runners like to stretch for almost the same amount of time as they have exercised; for others, stretching is a chore that they would prefer to avoid.

Why stretch?

You might think that running will give you strong legs, and it will up to a point, but if those legs lack flexibility it will not be long before you pick up an injury. To enable your muscles to perform at their peak, they must have a full range of motion, and that's where stretching comes in. Elongating your muscles after a run when they are warm will help to improve flexibility and promote circulation. Every run should end with a stretch.

When to stretch

Stretching and warming up are not the same thing yet it's common to see runners wildly stretching cold muscles at the start of a race. You're likely to injure yourself if you join them. Only ever stretch muscles when they are warm after a gentle run of at least 10 minutes. Your pre-run - and pre-race - strategy should be to complete a gentle warm up before you begin running harder, and leave the stretching till the finish when your muscles are warmed up.

10-minute stretches

The following five stretches should form the bare minimum that you do after your run. You do not

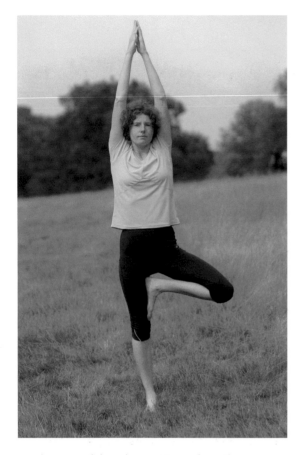

Many runners benefit from the added strength and flexibility that yoga and Pilates provide.

need any special equipment to perform them – you do not even need to sit down. In fact, you can do them anywhere, so there's no excuse to skip them.

Don't bounce

Never bounce when you are stretching. You should ease yourself gently into each position until you feel mild tension, and then hold the stretch for 10–20 seconds before relaxing. Repeat the stretch for another 10 seconds. You can increase the time if you feel comfortable.

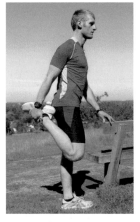

Quadriceps stretch
Stand up straight with your feet shoulder-width apart. Lift your right heel towards your bottom, taking care not to lock your left knee. To increase the stretch, gently push your right hip forward. Change legs and then repeat.

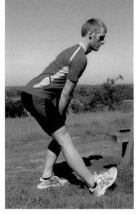

Hamstrings stretch
Stand with your feet parallel, about a foot apart. Keep your front leg straight and bend your back leg. Push your hips back and away from your front foot. You should feel a stretch in the hamstring of your straight leg. Change legs and then repeat on the other side.

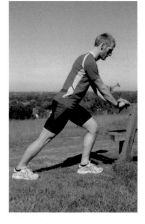

Calf stretch
Holding onto a support, such as a chair or desk, stand with your feet a stride-length apart. Your front knee should be bent and your back knee straight. Push your back heel into the floor to stretch your calf. To stretch your lower calf, bend your back knee towards the floor. Change legs and repeat the stretch.

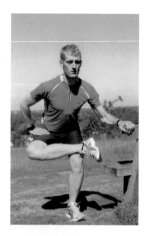

Glutes stretch

Stand with your feet shoulder-width apart. Place your right ankle across your left leg, just above the knee. Using a table or chair for support, drop your bottom to create a right angle with your left leg. You should feel a stretch in your right buttock. Change legs and repeat.

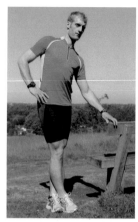

Hip stretch

Stand up straight with your right leg crossed over your left and the outsides of your feet together. Lean your body to the left, shifting your weight onto your left leg. Change legs and repeat. You can hold onto a chair (as shown above) or table for support if you wish.

Running technique

You now know what to do before and after a run, but what about during the run itself? Few people are taught how to run – it is just something that everyone learns to do in childhood. But how do you know if you are running correctly?

Finding a running style

Sit on a park bench near any popular running route and watch the style of each runner who passes you. You can guarantee that no two runners will ever look the same. Most will strike on the heel but some will land and push off on their toes without ever putting their heel down.

Everyone has a different running style, so you need to find out what works best for you. It is important that you feel relaxed and comfortable when you run – you can even nod your head like Paula Radcliffe if that feels good. Trying to change your natural running style can take years and is not something to attempt lightly, but a few subtle adjustments to your form could help you to run more easily and efficiently.

Run tall

Imagine that you have a string tied to the top of your head. Your head should be in line with your shoulders, with your hips directly underneath. Relax your upper body, from your shoulders down to your fingertips, and aim to keep your arms tucked in. By maintaining good posture when you're running, you will open up your lungs, allowing more air to be transported to where it's needed.

Look up

It can be tempting and sometimes necessary to look at your feet when you are running, but try to keep your focus on the horizon instead.

Running uphill

You will find it easier to conquer hills if you shorten your stride and slow your pace. Your level of effort should remain constant, rather than your pace.

Stride rate

You have decided that you want to crank up the pace a bit. To achieve this, you could take longer strides, but the best way to run faster is to quicken your leg turnover.

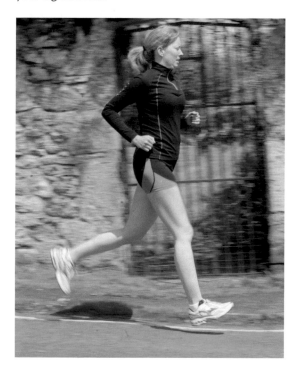

Running tall with your head held high will ensure that your lungs are always full of oxygen.

Assessing progress

Even if you have no aspirations to compete in a race, you might still be interested to know whether you're improving as a runner. Progress means different things to different people, but being a runner always means celebrating your achievements, no matter how insignificant they might seem to others.

must know

Explore your options
It's not just the steps you take in your running shoes that can help you progress as a runner. Other kinds of exercise can be just as useful. A weights programme, for example, will build muscle to enable you to run stronger for longer.

Progress pointers

If you no longer take walk breaks when you run, you're making progress. If you can run for longer than you were previously able to, you're making progress. If your resting heart rate is lower, you've lost weight or notice that your clothes feel a little looser, you're making progress. Even if you just feel better about yourself, you're making progress.

How to gauge improvement

While your goals are unique to you, a time will come when you might compare yourself to other runners. Here is a simple way to assess your progress without racing every weekend. Find a route that you know is roughly a mile – use a running track or measure it in your car or on your bike. After warming up, run the mile as fast as you can, then record your time. Repeat once a month: as the time it takes you to run the mile falls, you'll be able to gauge how your running is improving. If you don't make progress from one month to the next, don't get disheartened. Running improvements are never linear. One month you might feel great but record a slower time than another month when you feel tired but put in a better performance. Just focus on your next run.

Recovery

Recovery is the part of the training process that very few people understand. You need to build in rest days, as per the training schedules at the end of this book, rather than become obsessed with running every day and feeling guilty if you miss a day.

Rest is important

The improvements you make in your running will not follow a neat pattern, nor does it follow that piling on the miles makes you a better runner. You might not feel that your running is progressing if you are sorting out the garden or going for a bike ride with your kids, but the time you spend resting in between runs is one of the most important components of your new running regime.

Complete rest or some cross-training, such as cycling or swimming, will improve your running just as much as the tough run you did the day before. You might have had such a great run on Monday that you are tempted to go out again on Tuesday, but not allowing your body enough time to recover is the fastest way to become injured.

> **must know**
>
> **Time to adapt**
> Alternate hard and easy days to give your body time to adapt. Listen to your body and follow its message. If your legs feel heavy, don't run the next day. You do not have to stop exercising; just have a break from running until you feel that the spring's back in your step.

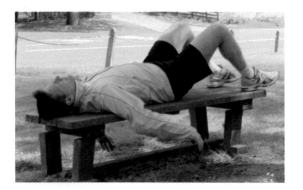

Don't risk burning out by going running every day – rest is just as important as training.

Running surfaces

Now that you know how to protect yourself from potential risks, you should also find out how to protect yourself from injury by training on a variety of different surfaces, which can affect your running in different ways.

Hard versus soft surfaces

If you have ever bounced a football on the road, then on a grass pitch, you will know that it bounces higher on the road. That's because a road is hard, and it returns most of the energy you put into it, bouncing the ball straight back up at you. A grass pitch is softer, absorbing your energy and killing the bounce. The same is true when your foot lands on a variety of different surfaces.

Pavements and roads

Hard roads and pavements will return the force of each footfall straight back into your legs. Every time your foot hits the ground, it lands with a force of three to four times your body weight. Even though they are often the most convenient option, try to limit the time that you train on roads to protect your body from the impact.

Grass

Grass is a wonderfully soft surface to run on, but, while you are less likely to become injured if you run on grass, there are still some pitfalls to watch out for. It can be easy to turn an ankle over on uneven ground, so place your feet carefully and look out for any bumps and hollows.

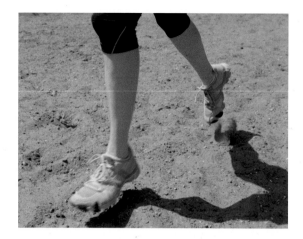

Training on different surfaces, such as sand, will help you to become a stronger runner.

Sand

Running on sand is a great way to strengthen your whole body because it forces you to work harder to balance and move forward. The dryer and softer the sand, the kinder it is to your legs, but it's also the hardest workout of all for a runner. If you are running on the beach, start off in the more compacted sand by the water's edge.

Trails

The varied terrain on off-road trails makes them the perfect surface for extended runs. Your muscles and joints will appreciate the forgiving terrain, and your mind will stay interested as you focus on leaping over a tree root or avoiding a rock.

Track

An artificial 400m running track is great for a speed session, but don't do all your long runs on one, unless there's no alternative. If you do, run in the outer lanes where the bends are not as tight and change direction regularly to avoid injury.

want to know more?

• Visit a specialist running shop to have your gait analysed. They will be able to advise you which running shoes best suit your style of running.
• To read hundreds of product reviews, or to add a review of your own, log on to: www.runnersworld.co.uk/gear
• Look out for a free shoe guide in *Runner's World* magazine four times a year.
• Find out more about running form at www.chirunning.com and www.posetech.com
• Find a local yoga class by visiting the British Wheel of Yoga website at: www.bwy.org.uk

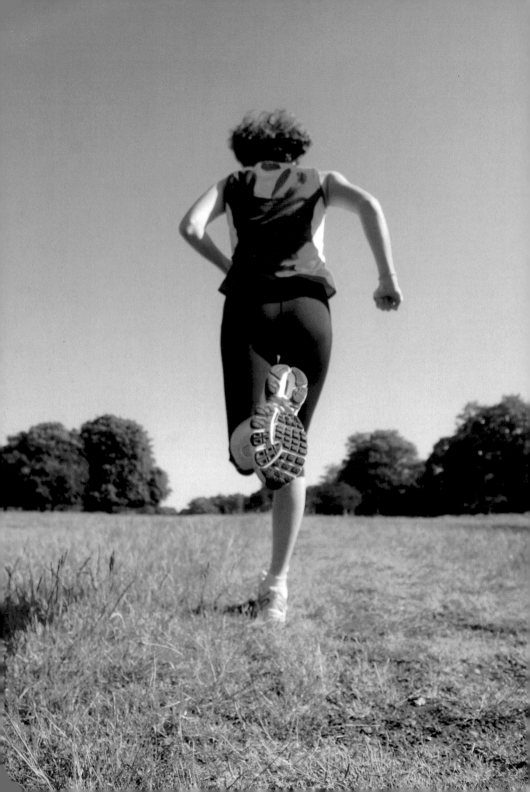

2 Basic training

Now that you are able to run for more than 30 minutes, it's time to explore the different ways you can train. Do you really need to run up hills, spend hours on your feet, or make regular visits to the track? In this section you can find out how to put together the perfect training week, why you need to make friends with fartlek and how to run hills the easy way as well as the essential training tools that no runner should be without.

Different types of training

There are as many reasons to run as there are runners. You may start running to lose weight, or you might decide that it's time to improve your fitness. Alternatively, you might run to escape a hectic family or working life, or you might want to take part in a race. Whatever the reason, choose your training regime carefully.

must know

Racing
There are thousands of races in the UK every year. Whether you want to join more than 750,000 women in a Race for Life 5K or run your first marathon, there's a race out there with your name on it. For a comprehensive guide to the races coming up in your area, see: www.runnersworld.co.uk/events

New kinds of running

When you can run confidently for half an hour or more, you might decide to explore new kinds of running. You may want to challenge yourself to run faster or for longer than you have done before, or you might just feel that your running routine needs more variety to freshen it up and keep you interested. When a friend persuades you that it's time to enter your first race, or you decide that the time has come to smash your 10K personal best, you need to know the different types of training you can adopt to reach your goal.

Running stronger for longer

If you have been heading out for three or four runs a week up to now, you will probably have noticed some improvements in both your speed and your endurance. Regular runs are a great way to enhance your stamina, but if you want to run stronger for longer, you will need a more focused training plan. There are several ways in which you can train that will help to build speed, stamina and mental toughness – all key weapons in every runner's arsenal – as well as injecting some healthy variety into your workouts.

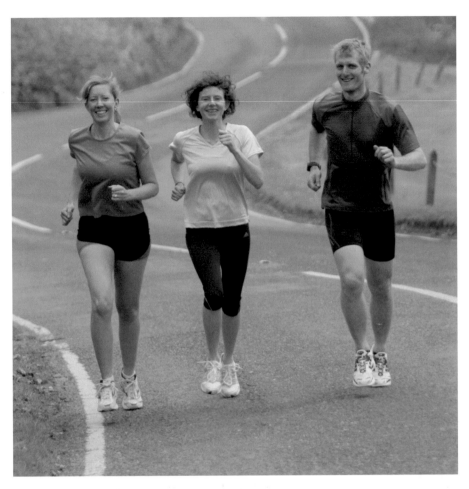

Train smart

The following pages explain the different types of
running that you can incorporate into your training
schedule. Depending on what you want to achieve,
you can run slow or fast, for short or long periods,
to build up speed, stamina or both. Try to include
a variety of sessions in your schedule, although
a sensible approach is to go easy on the speed and
hill work if you are new to running.

**Training with friends is one of
the best ways to ensure that you
never miss a run.**

Interval training

It's an old running adage that the only way to run faster is to run faster. That usually means incorporating some interval training, or speed work as it's often known, into your training programme.

Intervals

At their most basic, intervals are periods of hard effort broken up by periods of easier effort, which allow your body to recover. They teach your body how to cope with faster running, and condition your mind to push you out of your comfort zone.

When you run a fast-paced interval, your body relies on something called your anaerobic system to provide energy to your working muscles – you have probably experienced this as a burning sensation in your legs. It is caused by a build up of lactic acid, which is partially broken down as your body rebalances the supply of oxygen to your muscles when you slow your pace during the recovery.

Inject some speed

Running faster than you are accustomed to will encourage your body to create more oxygen-delivering capillaries and builds your tolerance to lactic acid, enabling you to run harder for longer periods before experiencing the burning sensation. If you want to inject some speed into your running, a weekly interval session will teach your body to run more quickly. It's also a great way to build endurance and avoid injury by giving you an intense workout over a relatively short period. Join up with friends or a group to make the session more fun.

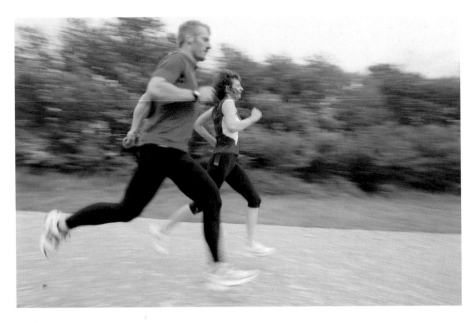

Try this

If you are training for a marathon, you might choose to run longer intervals at a slower pace than if you were training for a shorter race, such as a 5K. When training for a half-marathon or marathon, try to run hard for five minutes, jog for two, and repeat up to four times. If you're training for a shorter race, such as a 5K or 10K, running a pyramid is a classic interval session. Run 200m, 400m, 800m, 400m, 200m with two minutes' rest between each interval. Try to run on a forgiving surface, such as a football pitch or dirt trail, and limit interval training to one session a week. If you have access to a running track, a great interval session is to run hard on the straights and jog to recover on the bends. These short intervals mean you should be able to keep going for longer as lactic acid won't have time to build up in your legs. Start with five laps.

Pick up the pace every now and then when you're out running.

must know

Distance and pace
Many runners like to complete their speedier sessions with friends or at a club. Most clubs have weekly interval sessions where you'll be placed with runners of a similar ability. If you train alone, a treadmill is a great way to control distance and pace during interval sessions.

Fartlek

The term 'fartlek' is derived from a Swedish word meaning speed play. It is a flexible and fun way to interval train and can be done on any terrain and over any distance.

must know

Holiday running
You might not feel like running when you are on holiday but you can easily fit in some short, sharp efforts as you explore the local area. You can try using your surroundings on a fartlek run, perhaps by speeding up and slowing down between lamp posts at the sea front, or by catching up with other runners whom you see ahead of you.

How fartlek works

There is no set formula: you determine the intensity that you run periods of effort – when the pace should be higher than your regular training – and how long you want to ease back for in between to recover. Fartlek sessions are a good way to prepare for races as they train your aerobic and anaerobic systems, equipping you to speed up or slow down over difficult terrain, or in line with changes of pace set by an opponent. The hard efforts should make up at least 50 per cent of the distance covered, and include one section of at least 600m at greater-than-race pace. Include one fartlek session in your weekly schedule.

Try this

Fartlek sessions are less structured than interval sessions, and they are designed to be more fun. In fact, they are great to run with a friend or with a group of runners. Next time you're running with a few friends, run in a line taking it in turns to choose the length and intensity of a period of effort and recovery. If you're on your own, spice up a fartlek session by putting in a fast burst every time you see a red car, for example, or between telegraph poles. Just because you're speeding up doesn't mean your running style should fall apart. Try to make each step fluid and relaxed even when you turn up the pace.

Opposite: Create your own fartlek session by using areas of light and shade to vary your pace.

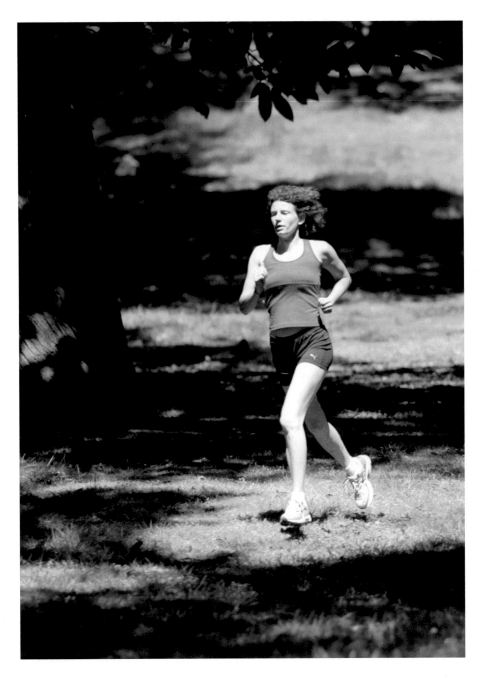

Tempo runs

Tempo runs, or threshold runs as they are sometimes known, are another way to teach your body to run fast before fatigue sets in. There are two kinds of tempo run – one long controlled run of up to about five miles and long interval runs of about a mile with short recoveries.

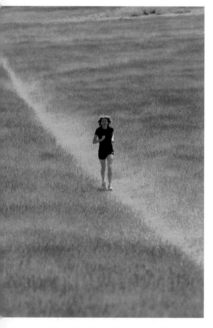

Run hard sessions on tracks or grass to protect against injury.

A sustainable pace

You should aim to run for at least 20 minutes at a pace that is a hard effort but is still sustainable evenly for the duration. It might feel easy at the start, but you need to hold the pace throughout.

Finding the right pace can be one of the trickiest parts of tempo running, but with a little trial and error you will come up with a pace that leaves you feeling that you have put in the maximum effort by the time you finish the session. Tempo runs are supposed to be tough, but that does not mean you put in so much effort that you collapse at the end. All speed work – including intervals and fartlek – is about sustained effort rather than all-out effort, so it's a good idea to err on the side of caution the first few times you run a session.

Try this

Measure a lap of three to four miles. You're going to use this loop every week to gauge your progress. Run the lap at a hard but controlled pace and note your time. Next week, see if you can run a little faster at the same effort. Tempo runs should make up no more than 15 per cent of your total weekly mileage, so limit these sessions to one per week.

Hill running

Hill running is a great way of building up your strength and speed without forcing you to run too fast. It is also a good session to run on your own because the hill will ensure that you have enough of a challenge. Running hills also builds your mental confidence which carries over into other areas of your running.

Training on hills

Training on the flat is fine when you're starting out, but the further you run the more likely you are to encounter hills, so at some point you have to start training on them. Begin with a hilly workout every other week to give your body the chance to adapt to the new stresses you are placing on it, then build up gradually until you're doing a regular weekly session.

Try this

Find a long incline that is not too steep and extends for at least 200-300m. Run up it, using your arms to power you forwards and maintaining high knees. Walk back down to the start and repeat. You may only be able to manage one or two ascents and recoveries to begin with, but aim to build this up to five ascents after four weeks.

Adapt your style

It is easier to tackle hills if you shorten your stride when the gradient rises. Pump your arms to provide momentum on uphill runs; use them for balance when you're picking up speed on the descents. You can lengthen your stride a little downhill but do not overdo it or you may start to lose control.

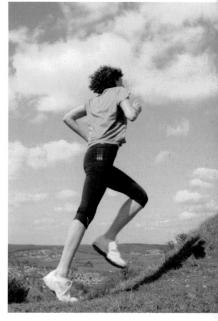

Hill running will make you a stronger, faster runner.

Long runs

If you join a club or talk to other runners before a race, you will hear them discuss their weekly long runs with reverence. Long runs are the backbone of endurance training and an essential element in every training schedule from the 5K up to ultra marathons.

must know

Why run long?
Long runs do not just deliver physical benefits; they are a fantastic psychological boost, too. If you're training for a marathon, knowing that you're capable of running 20 miles in training will give you the confidence that you need to go the distance on race day. Long runs encourage your body to burn a greater portion of its fat as fuel, sparing the glycogen in your muscles and decreasing your risk of 'hitting the wall' (see page 135).

The key to success

There are two elements to successful long runs: the pace and the mind set. You should try to find a pace that is comfortably sustainable for the entire run. If you are running with someone, you should be able to carry on a conversation; if you are on your own, you should not be struggling for breath.

Many people do their long runs by time rather than by distance, which makes it easier to adjust your mind set to how long you are going to be out, whether it's 30 minutes or two hours. As you are going to be out running for some time, it is very important that you find a place to run that you enjoy being in – this is not a session to do on a treadmill or on crowded city pavements.

Try this
Run at an easy, even pace, with the first and last 10 minutes at the same pace. Build up the long run gradually to your target, increasing it by no more than 15 minutes per week. Drink regularly throughout the run, and if you are going to be running for 90 minutes or more, you should take on board some food as well. Give yourself a rest every fourth week and always precede and follow your long run day with an easy day or a complete rest.

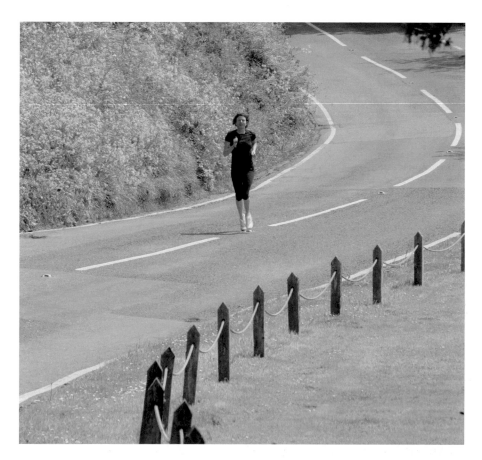

Your pace should be much slower on your long runs than in any other part of your training. That said, it is still okay to slow down even more and walk if you encounter a hill, for example, or if you are tired from running into a headwind.

Long runs are a key element of endurance training.

In good company

On your first few long runs it's a good idea to run with a friend or ask someone to keep you company on a bike. They can hand you drinks and snacks or offer encouragement if you hit a tough patch.

Training tools

Simplicity is a large part of running's appeal, but a little technology can help you move your training to another level. Here are some useful training aids and gadgets which you might consider.

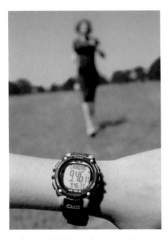

A stopwatch is a great tool for assessing your progress.

Running watch

The simplest – and a completely objective – way to judge your progress is to time yourself regularly over a known distance. A good running watch should have a stopwatch and a multiple lap counter to record miles, laps or intervals during a long training session or race. A model with a 50-lap counter should satisfy most runners' needs.

Heart rate monitor

The next step up from a watch, the heart rate monitor (HRM) combines a chest strap, which monitors your heart rate, and a wristwatch, which receives the information the chest strap transmits. Training by heart rate allows you to personalize every session, putting in the appropriate amount of effort for how your body feels on that day. A basic HRM provides a constant heart rate read-out and an ability to set high and low parameters to ensure you train in the correct heart rate zone. Information from more advanced models can be downloaded to a computer to analyse every session in detail.

Speed and distance monitor

The speed and distance monitor (SDM) is the most recent addition to the technology market and it uses GPS technology to record your speed, distance and pace accurately. An alternative system uses a measuring device that fits on your shoe and provides much the same information to an accompanying wristwatch. All SDMs also have basic stopwatch functions and some offer HRM alternatives.

Treadmills

This piece of indoor exercise equipment might not seem an obvious training tool but many runners use treadmills for precision speed and hill sessions, using their pace, distance or gradient features to run at set intervals. In simple terms, you can run any session that you run outside on a treadmill. When you're travelling for work and the only option is the treadmill in the hotel gym, or the cold and icy weather prevents you training outside, running on a treadmill means you need never miss a workout.

Belting along

Some runners find treadmill training monotonous, so next time you realize that you've looked at the stopwatch three times in the last minute, try these tips to beat the boredom. Run your hard interval sessions on a treadmill – you will be putting in so much effort that you won't notice the time tick by. Use the time you are on the treadmill to catch up on the day's news, listen to the album you just bought or chat to your neighbour. Concentrate on your running form: the treadmill will force you to run at an even pace, so take the opportunity to identify areas of your style that you might be able to improve. Anything from picking your feet up a little quicker to holding your shoulders further back can make a difference.

must know

Treadmills
Don't train exclusively on a treadmill – the action of running on a moving belt is slightly different from moving over solid ground. You should set the treadmill to a one per cent gradient to compensate for different weather conditions, both indoors and outdoors.

Planning your training

Running every other day, or when you feel like it, is a great strategy when you are new to running, but when the time comes to push yourself a little harder, you will need a plan.

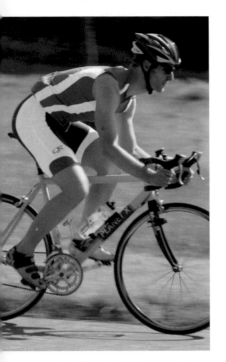

Feel like a break from running? Head out on your bike instead.

The perfect training week

Striking a balance between hard and easy sessions and training and recovery are the keys to the perfect training week. Once you have decided what the essential ingredients will be, you can work out how to fit them into your schedule. Most runners plan their long run for the weekend, for example, when they are home from work and there are fewer pressures on their time.

Planning your week

When you are deciding on what sort of training you want to fit into the coming training week, you might want to include the following:
- An interval session or tempo run, or both.
- An off-road long run.
- One complete day of rest.
- A cross-training session, such as swimming or cycling.

   It is always a good idea to aim to alternate your hard days with easy days. Remember that recovery does not necessarily mean a night spread out on the sofa catching up on your favourite soap opera. You can be more positive and go for a swim in the local pool, venture out for a bike ride with your children, or even just run more slowly than you would usually train.

Your training year

Planning your training year is just an extension of this weekly balance. You cannot expect to train hard all the year round, so ideally you should choose two or three goals and then focus on achieving them at different points in the year.

For example, if you decide that you are going to run a spring marathon, you will know that in the months leading up to the big race you will need to dedicate more time to training than usual. With this in mind, you should work out whether that will be possible with all your other work, social and family commitments at that time of year.

You may find that realizing your goal will not be possible within the time you have available, so you will need to revise your training plan. Remember that taking a break between periods of hard training will allow you to recover physically and mentally.

must know

Set a SMART goal
Deciding in January that you want to end the year by 'running faster' or 'weighing less' is great, but you are much more likely to achieve your target if you set a SMART goal. This means it should be Specific, Measurable, Achievable, Realistic and Timed. For example, you want to run your local Race for Life 5K in three months' time in under 30 minutes by training three times a week.

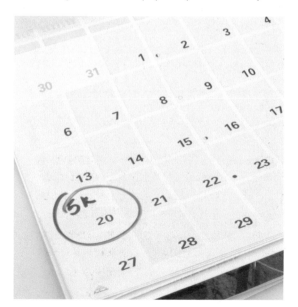

At the start of the year plan a few races that you'd like to tackle in the coming months. You can use races instead of training, too. Instead of a long run when you're marathon training, for example, why not enter a race instead?

must know

Training diaries

A training diary can reveal the successes and failures of training, helping you to develop strategies to improve your running. You might discover that you picked up an injury when you increased your weekly mileage suddenly, or that you did not give yourself enough rest before a race to perform well. You'll also be able to look back at your training when you've done well in a race and adopt any successful strategies again. Keeping a training diary can act as motivation, too. You don't want to see a blank page, so you're more likely to go for a run. When writing your diary, you should try to include the following.

Training diaries
Whether you write in a journal, scribble on a calendar, use a special computer programme or start a blog online to log your workouts, a training diary will only become a useful training tool if you complete it every time you run. Try to get into the habit of filling in the details as soon as you return from training. You will be able to use them to analyse past successes and failures and plan for the future.

Resting heart rate

When you wake up every morning, take your pulse before you get out of bed and make a note of it. With improved fitness, your resting pulse rate will fall. An elevated heart rate could be a sign that you're training too hard without giving yourself enough time to recover, or that you are coming down with a cold or virus.

Heart rate during training

Measuring your heart rate during a run can also indicate improved fitness. Since heart rate can reflect the amount of effort you are putting in, if you complete an identical route twice in the same time, but with a lower heart rate, you're becoming fitter.

Time on your feet and distance covered

Never increase the duration you run for by more than 10 per cent in a week. Likewise, never increase the distance you run by more than 10 per cent in a week.

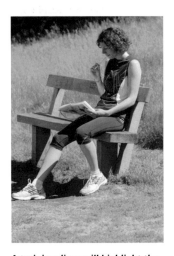

A training diary will highlight the strategies that work for you.

Shoe log

Record how many miles you have run in a particular pair of running shoes – their average effective life is about 500 miles. When your shoes reach this mileage, you should consider replacing them.

Time of day

Do you find getting up early to go for a run harder than completing a marathon? Some people just don't seem to be good at running early in the day. There's scientific evidence to suggest that you might find it easier to run at certain times of day. Keep track of how easy your run feels and the time of day at which you run, and you might discover what time suits you best.

Weather conditions

The weather can influence your running in a variety of ways. You might feel you have put in a lot of effort to run slowly when it's hot or humid. Equally, the cold weather can make running seem more difficult. If your times are slower, it could be nothing more than having to work harder to beat the elements.

Running surface

By training on different surfaces – road, grass or even sand – you'll give your body a chance to adapt. If you run on roads all the time, you might become injured because it's hard on your body.

How did you feel?

Don't become a slave to the numbers you record in your diary; how you felt can be as important as how far you ran. You may feel tired because you're having too many late nights or working too hard.

want to know more?

• One of the best ways to do interval training is as part of a group. To find your nearest running club, try the excellent 'club search' facility on the UK Athletics website. Just log on to: www.ukathletics.net and click on 'clubs'.
• Having trouble with your long runs or can't motivate yourself to do a weekly interval session? Find out how other runners approach their training by logging on to the *Runner's World* magazine website at: www.runnersworld.co.uk and click on 'forums'.
• Create an online training diary at: www.blogger.com

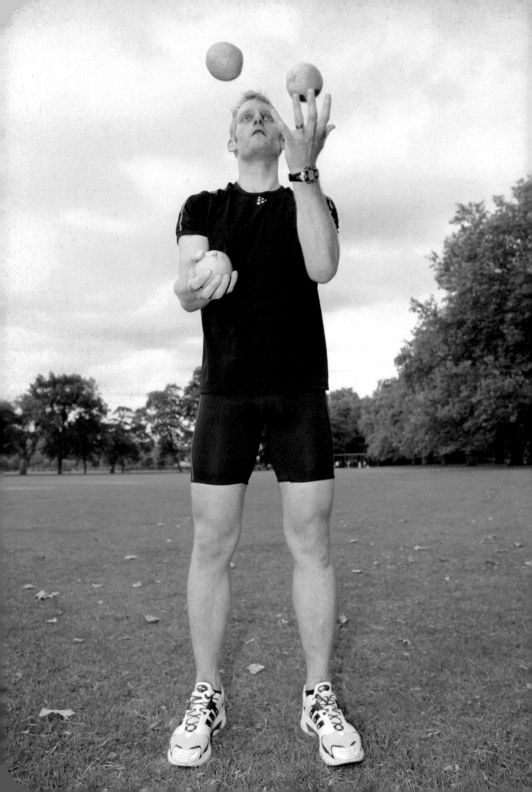

3 The basics of sports nutrition

Good nutrition alone will not make you a great runner, but it is part of the overall package that will enable you to reach your full potential. A plate of pasta before every run isn't enough to guarantee energy but a healthy, balanced diet combined with your new running routine will allow you to become the best runner you can be. From fats and fluids to carbohydrate, protein and fruit and vegetables, here's what to eat and drink before, during and after training.

Basic nutrition

Think of your body as an engine, and the food you consume as the fuel. If you have aspirations for your engine to perform at its highest level, you need to be careful about the fuel you put into it. A great engine with low-performance fuel will struggle to run smoothly. So it is with your body and food.

must know

How much do I need?
To work out exactly how many grams of carbohydrate to put away every day, just multiply your weight in kilograms by seven. So, if you weigh 70kg, for example, your daily diet should include 70 x 7 = 490g of carbohydrate.

You are what you eat

You need food to live and to run. The food itself will not make you a good or a fast runner – that's down to a combination of natural talent and training – but it can help you to train more efficiently, to recover more quickly and also to run to your full potential. Anyone who is serious about their running should also pay attention to the food they eat. That does not mean you have to live an alcohol-free life of low-fat pasta dinners and protein shakes, but it does mean that you should have at least a basic grasp of nutritional principles.

The basics

All food is made up of a combination of protein, fat and carbohydrate. Each of these nutrients provides a certain quantity of energy when it is broken down by your body: a gram of fat provides nine calories of energy, whereas a gram of carbohydrate or protein delivers four calories.

On an average day, a sedentary 70kg man would burn 2,500 calories, whereas an average 55kg woman would burn only 1,900 calories. Each would need to consume the same number of food calories to maintain their body weight. If you have a deficit between what you take in and what your body burns, you will lose weight, but if you eat more than the calories you are burning then you will gain weight. Running or any form of exercise increases the number of calories your body burns at the rate of approximately 100 calories per mile. Consequently, the main concern for most runners is that they have enough readily available energy to run the speeds and distances they want to without fatigue. It's therefore important to understand how your body uses and stores each nutrient.

Include a colourful variety of fruit and vegetables in your diet.

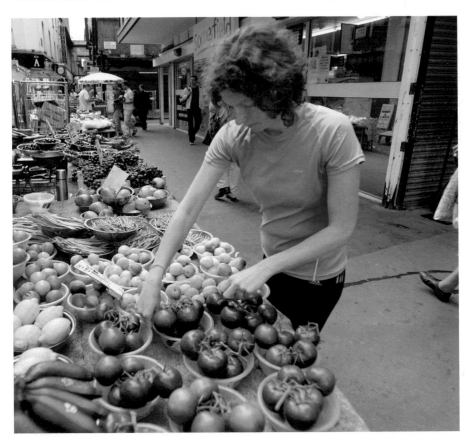

Carbohydrates

Carbohydrate is the body's primary source of readily available fuel and should form a significant part of every runner's diet. Stored as glycogen in the muscles and liver, it is the fuel your body burns first when you start running, and the one it relies upon for prolonged intensive exercise. The big down-side of carbohydrate is that your body can only store a limited supply of it, around 1,600 calories' worth.

Carbohydrates are classed as simple or complex, depending on their chemical structure. Simple carbohydrates consist of one or two sugar molecules, such as glucose, sucrose, fructose and lactose, while complex carbohydrates include starches and fibres and are made up of much larger molecules.

Always start the day with a healthy breakfast that includes some carbohydrate.

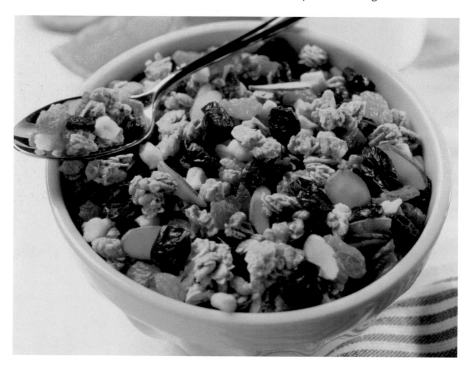

In reality, most foods will contain both simple and complex carbohydrates.

The most helpful way to measure the usefulness of carbohydrates to the runner, is to consider how quickly certain foods can enter the blood stream. The glycaemic index (GI) is a number that is given to carbohydrate-rich food based on the average increase in blood glucose levels after consumption. Most foods fall between 20 and 100. A food with a high GI, such as a sugary sports drink, will produce a rapid rise in your blood sugar levels. A low GI food, such as porridge or pasta, will produce a less rapid rise, resulting in a more sustained release of energy.

Is it possible to eat too many carbs?

Your new exercise regime may have you reaching for the pasta to fuel up before every run, but you will still need to consider your overall calorie intake. Since your body can only store so much carbohydrate, any surplus that you are not using will be converted and stored in your fat reserves, meaning you will put on weight. Overeating is overeating, whether it's carbohydrate, fat or protein that you're consuming. You might have heard that before a marathon or other endurance event athletes attempt to 'carbo load'. This means they start the race with as much stored muscle glycogen – which fuels the effort – as possible. There is some debate among sports nutritionists about the best ways to carbo load but a good general rule is to consume a diet that is high in carbohydrate, protein, vitamins and minerals, combined with plenty of fluids, in the two to three days leading up to the event, and to rest completely the day before you race.

must know

Top 10 carbs
- Brown rice
- Wholemeal pasta
- Oats/porridge
- Whole-grain cereals
- Whole-wheat bread
- Potatoes
- Bagels
- Bananas
- Energy bars
- Milkshakes

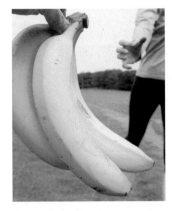

Bananas are a handy source of energy for runners.

must know

How much do I need?
To work out how much
protein to include in
your daily diet, multiply
your weight in kilograms
by 1.3. This will give you
the number of grams of
protein you should eat
every day. So, if you
weigh 70kg, multiply
70 x 1.3 = 91g protein.

Protein

Protein is not usually an important source of
energy. Its most important role in your diet is to
repair muscles and other tissues that are damaged
during training. The body breaks protein down into
one of 20 amino acids which not only rebuild tissue
but also help cells to transport oxygen round the
body and create hormones, such as adrenalin.
Your body would rather use carbohydrate to create
energy, but when your liver and muscle glycogen
stores are empty – perhaps towards the end of
a long run or a bike ride – protein may be used as
an alternative source of energy, but still in relatively
small proportions.

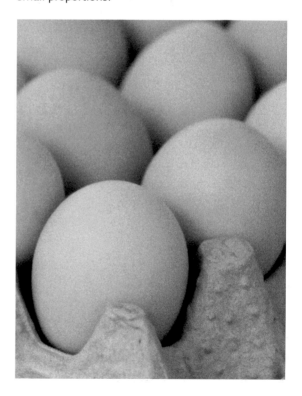

Eggs are a great source of
protein, as well as being low in
saturated fat and calories. If
you're vegetarian, choose eggs
fortified with omega-3.

Your recovery window

Many recent studies have demonstrated that protein is essential for our short-term recovery, too. By combining carbohydrate and protein in a post-run snack, you will help your body to recover rapidly and be ready for your next training session. Aim to eat a snack, such as a glass of milk, a bagel with peanut butter, or a turkey sandwich, within 20 minutes of finishing a training session.

Strong stuff

If you are trying to put on muscle by including resistance exercises in your training schedule, your protein requirements will be higher still. Aim to eat 1.6 grams of protein per kilogram of body weight.

Protein supplements

Your daily balanced diet should include enough protein, but if you think you might be struggling to eat an adequate amount, then you could try taking a protein supplement. These are generally powders that are mixed with milk to create a flavoured drink which is similar to a milkshake. These drinks are popular post-training to aid recovery.

Protein pitfalls

Do not be tempted to limit your protein intake to eating a juicy steak every evening. Red meat is a great source of protein, but it can also be quite high in saturated fat. So swap the steak for a slice of salmon or tuna. They are a great source of protein *and* heart-healthy oils that lower your risk of heart disease. Dairy products also provide protein but be sure to choose low-fat versions.

must know

Top 10 proteins
- Lean meat, e.g. beef
- Poultry, including turkey, chicken and ostrich
- Eggs
- Skimmed milk
- Cottage cheese
- Low-fat fruit yoghurt
- Oily fish, e.g. salmon and tuna
- Nuts
- Tofu
- Beans

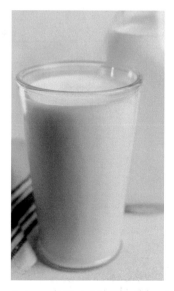

A glass of milk drunk after a run combines carbohydrate and protein to help you recover.

must know

Types of fat
It's the type of fat you eat, rather than the amount you consume, that's most important. The Mediterranean diet, for example, is high in fats yet people who eat it tend to be less at risk from heart disease.

Fats

Fat is your body's most abundant source of energy. We all have enough, stored either around the organs or beneath the skin, to keep us running for over 1,000 miles. Unfortunately, we would have to cover those miles very slowly to use stored fat as energy, because as soon as you move up into a slow run, your body switches to carbohydrate as its primary fuel source. Generally speaking, the harder or faster you run, the greater the proportion of carbohydrate and the lower the proportion of fat your body uses.

However, all fats are not equal. There are good and bad fats as well as fats that fall somewhere in between. Fat is an essential part of a runner's diet, but it is the type of fat rather than the overall amount that you eat which is the key.

Good fats

Monounsaturated fats contain lower levels of 'bad' (LDL) cholesterol, and raise 'good' (HDL) cholesterol. The good cholesterol keeps your arteries clean and protects against heart disease. Aim to include monounsaturated fats in your diet by eating two portions of oily fish every week. Polyunsaturated fats are usually liquid at room temperature and include vegetable oils, such as sunflower oil. They are halfway between monounsaturated and saturated fats.

Bad fats

Saturated fats raise levels of 'bad' (LDL) cholesterol in the blood, and have been linked to a higher risk of heart disease and stroke. They are mostly animal fats and tend to have a waxy or buttery consistency at room temperature. Common sources include red meat, poultry, butter and full-fat milk.

Transfats

These are created by adding hydrogen to vegetable oil – to make it more solid and less likely to turn rancid. This is a useful process for the baked goods industry to increase a product's shelf life but bad news for you. Transfats raise your levels of bad cholesterol, fur up arteries, and have even been linked to Alzheimer's disease because they may block blood flow to the brain. If you see the words 'hydrogenated vegetable oil' in a list of a product's ingredients, put the packet down immediately and look for a healthier option.

must know

Top 10 healthy fats
- Avocado
- Olive oil
- Peanut butter
- Almonds
- Pumpkin seeds
- Mackerel
- Flaxseed oil
- Walnuts
- Tofu
- Fortified eggs

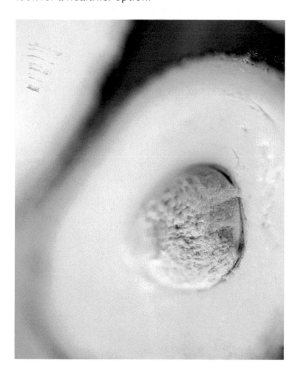

Avocados contain mostly monounsaturated fat, which has been shown to lower cholesterol. They are also packed with nutrients, including vitamin E and beta carotene, two powerful antioxidants.

Hydration

Just as your body needs food for fuel, it needs water to function. Water is the largest constituent in the human body, making up 60 per cent of your total body weight. It is crucial for carrying food, eliminating waste, regulating temperature, cushioning and lubricating joints, and maintaining blood volume and pressure.

must know

Sweating
Everyone sweats at a different rate, and the length and intensity of any run, plus the temperature, will affect how much you sweat. The best way to assess your fluid loss, and thus how much you need to drink, is to weigh yourself before and after a run. A weight loss of 1kg (2lb) requires a fluid replacement of 1 litre (1¾ pints), but many sports nutritionists recommend replacing one-and-a-half times the amount of fluid lost.

Your body needs water

The water demands placed on your body increase when you run because you start to lose fluid, mostly through sweating. Your body has a finely tuned thermostat that tries to keep your core temperature between 37 and 38°C to protect your heart and other vital organs. The extra energy produced when you run creates a lot of excess heat that has to be removed, and sweating is the most efficient way to do this.

You can't stop your body from sweating because it is a natural process. The faster and longer you run and the higher the air temperature, the more you sweat and the more fluid you lose. If you do not replace it, you run the risk of becoming dehydrated which can not only affect your performance but can also damage your health. Just a two per cent loss of body weight through fluid loss can lead to as much as a 20 per cent drop in your performance. Fortunately, it's quite an easy problem to rectify.

Before you run
To be well hydrated, drink 500ml (18fl oz) fluid two hours before running, e.g. water, a carbohydrate-based sports drink or diluted fruit juice. Drink 150ml (5fl oz) fluid just before you head out of the door.

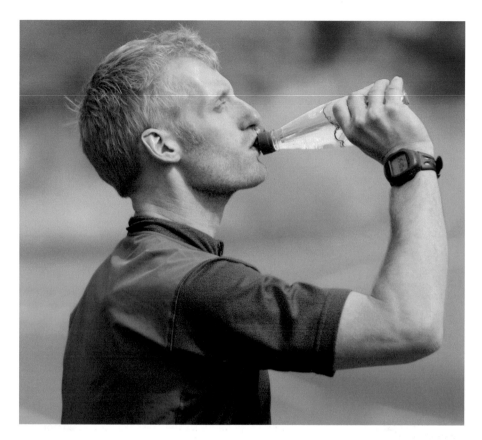

During a run

Running is literally thirsty work. The harder or faster you run, the more you need to drink to limit the potential side effects of dehydration. Current guidelines recommend drinking anything from 300ml (10fl oz) to 800ml (28fl oz) of fluids per hour when you are exercising. A good rule of thumb is to drink when you're thirsty.

Experiment in training and races with different amounts of fluid. This will help you to establish how your body responds to dehydration and also to find out what works best for you.

You should aim to start every run well hydrated. Aim to drink 500ml (18fl oz) of water or a sports drink two hours before the start of a race.

What should you drink?

For any run lasting less than an hour, water is your best fluid replacement choice. It is primarily what your body is losing through sweat and what it needs to replace, so you can't go wrong by drinking water. However, if you have been running hard for more than an hour, a drink containing simple sugar or a more complex form of carbohydrate and sodium (most branded sports drinks contain these) is likely to speed up your recovery compared with plain water.

This is because sports drinks which contain carbohydrate increase water absorption into your bloodstream, which is great news when you are sweating heavily. Flavoured sports drinks beat water on taste: because they taste good, you're more likely to drink them than water and thus more likely to stay hydrated. Diluted fruit juice (half and half with water) is also a good choice. Drinking water on its own has been shown to dilute the sodium in your blood, thereby reducing your urge to drink before you are fully hydrated.

Remember to drink more fluids when you run in hot weather.

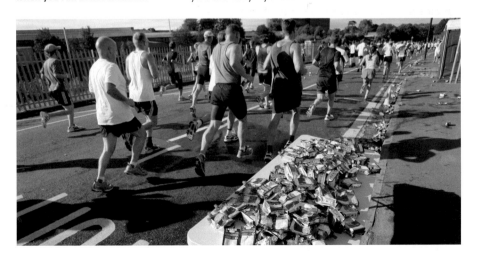

Weather

Hot, humid conditions will raise your temperature and increase the rate that you sweat, so you must consume extra fluid. Nor should you underestimate your fluid losses on wet or windy days. Wind chill can lead to rapid sweat evaporation, giving you the false impression that you are not losing much fluid.

Running in the cold can blunt your thirst, and wearing several layers of clothing can increase your temperature as well as sweat loss. Even if you don't feel hot and sweaty, dehydration is a risk, so try to make drinking before, during and after a run a habit.

Caffeine

There's no need to forgo your morning cup of tea or espresso before you run. Some runners steer clear of caffeine, believing it to have a diuretic effect during exercise, but numerous studies have shown that this is a myth: caffeine taken before a run will not dehydrate you or have a negative effect on your performance. At rest, however, drinks containing caffeine may make you go to the toilet more often. One study showed that a daily caffeine intake of up to 300mg produced no greater urine loss than water.

Alcohol

Having an espresso before your run won't do you any harm but drinking alcohol the night before could have a negative impact. Alcohol provides no useable energy and is also a mild diuretic. Taken in moderation, it should not be a major problem, but if you do opt for a glass of wine or beer the night before a run, aim to drink plenty of water, too, especially if the weather is hot.

must know

Improved performance
Drinks containing caffeine are actually likely to improve your performance. Studies suggest that a shot of caffeine before a run could improve your endurance by as much as 30 per cent.

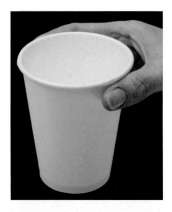

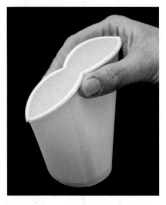

When you are handed a cup of water to drink during a race, just pinch the sides together to create a drinking spout.

Opposite: Drink a little at every drinks station you pass in a race.

How to drink on the run

Drinking on the run is an essential skill. You can train yourself to run with a reasonably full stomach by taking frequent small sips rather than gulping down a pint of fluid at one or two stops. If you don't want to carry a water bottle, plan a circuit around your home and stop off every time you pass to grab a drink, or practise drinking every few miles when you're on the treadmill.

Drinking in races

Many races provide bottled water and carbohydrate drinks, for easy drinking on the move, but if you're handed a paper cup, pinch the sides together to create a drinking spout. If you can't drink and run at the same time, slow down or walk a few steps while you take fluid on board; it's false economy not to drink.

must know

Hyponatraemia
With more people running marathons and completing them more slowly, hyponatraemia is a potential health danger. When runners drink too much water, especially over a prolonged period, the sodium in the body may become diluted. In its mild form, this causes bloating and nausea, but in a few rare cases it can lead to brain seizure and death. Women are more at risk as they're smaller and less muscular than men, so they sweat less and need to drink up to 30 per cent less. If you're running for more than four hours, be guided by thirst and use a sports drink that contains sodium instead of water.

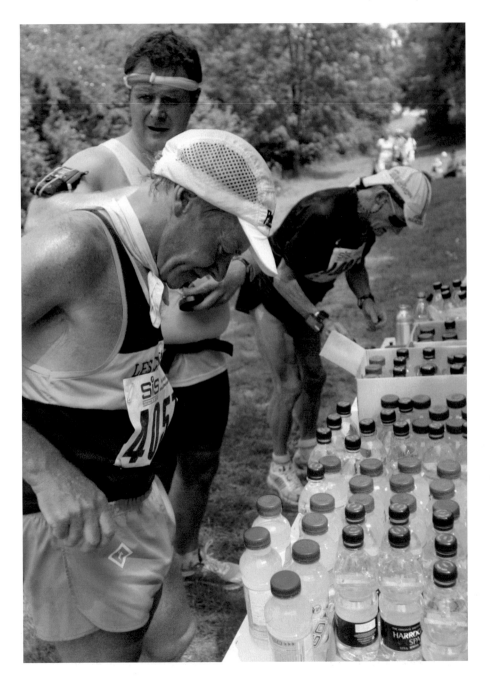

Hydration test
To find out whether you are dehydrated, check the colour of your urine as soon as you wake up. If you're well hydrated, it should be a pale yellow straw colour. If it's darker, you should be drinking more. Don't perform this test after taking a vitamin supplement as it can affect the colour of your urine. Opinion varies about how much water you need to drink every day, but the Food Standards Agency recommends six to eight 250ml (8fl oz) glasses.

Sports drinks

Sports drinks used to be simple – it was a choice of plain water or flavoured water, both of which could keep you hydrated but little else. Now there are specially formulated 'sports drinks' that will help you before, during or after your run – there are drinks that will make you more alert or even offer an alternative to a meal, and there is at least one product that claims to make you stronger while you are sleeping.

It's easy to be confused about what's on offer, particularly when the labels, such as sport, energy, carbohydrate, isotonic, etc., are so confusing. So here's a guide to understanding the sports drink market together with what to drink and when.

Understanding the label
Don't read too much into the label, as there is little consistency with terminology and its meaning. The role of today's sports drink (we'll ignore protein drinks for the moment) is two-fold: to replace fluid and electrolytes lost through sweating and to put back or top up the body's carbohydrate reserves. How well a drink fulfils each role depends on the concentration of carbohydrate it contains, which is something you can see on the label of a pre-mixed drink and need to think about when you are mixing your own.

If the carbohydrate is more than 10 per cent of the drink, it will slow down the rate at which your body can absorb the fluid and therefore use it to replace that lost through sweating.

If rehydration is your main priority, look for a drink that is hypotonic, i.e. one that is more dilute than

Opposite: Learning how to eat and drink on the run is an invaluable skill for runners.

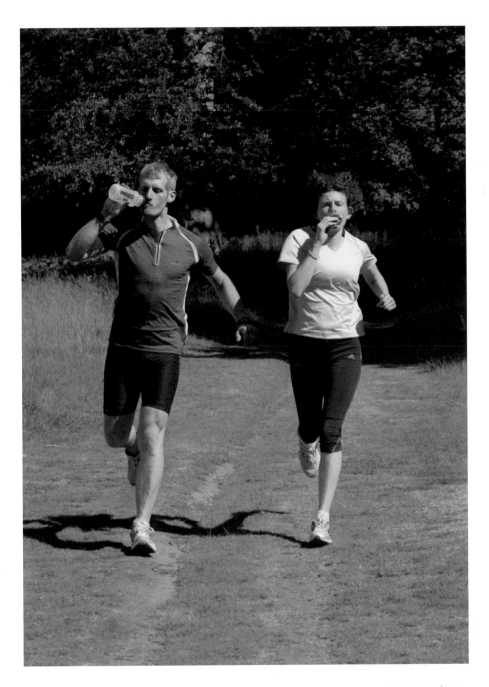

must know

The right sports drink
• **Run of less than 30 minutes: nothing or water**
• **Gentle-steady run up to 1 hour: water**
• **High-intensity run up to 1 hour: hypotonic or isotonic sports drink**
• **High-intensity run of more than 1 hour: hypotonic or isotonic sports drink**

your body fluids, such as orange squash or diluted fruit juices, because your body can absorb it quicker than plain water. Isotonic drinks have the same concentration of particles as your body. Popular brands can be absorbed as fast as water while also providing some additional fuel.

Drinks that are more concentrated than body fluids are hypertonic and will slow down the rate of absorption of fluid and would include neat fruit juices and many fizzy drinks.

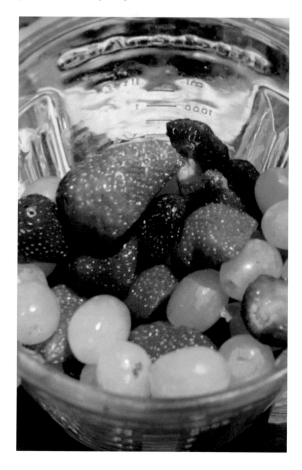

Enjoy a post-run smoothie to rehydrate and recover after a training session. A blend of fruit, milk and yoghurt will provide the perfect combination of nutrients, carbohydrate and protein.

Protein drinks

If you spend enough time in health food stores or sports shops you will come across protein drinks, which offer a heavy dose of carbohydrate and protein as a recovery drink. Most recreational runners will find that there is enough protein in their normal diet to ignore these drinks.

Gels

Gels are a relatively recent addition to the sports nutrition market and are less of a drink but more a concentrated shot of carbohydrate. They can not only supplement your drinks but also offer an easy, transportable way of eating on the run during long endurance runs and races. In fact, many people use gels and water rather than worrying about a particular carbohydrate drink.

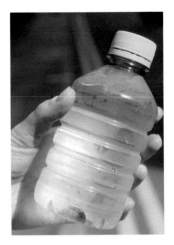

On runs of up to one hour, drink water to rehydrate.

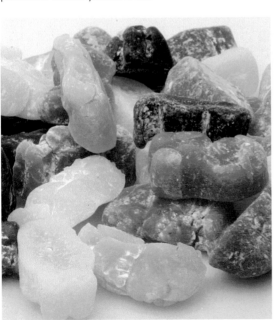

Gels are a handy way to consume carbohydrate during a race or training run. Wash them down with water and you will stay hydrated, too. An alternative to sports gels is to eat some jelly baby sweets.

The perfect runner's diet

A food pyramid is a great way to visualize how much you should be eating of the essential food groups. The latest research from the United States suggests that the UK's dietary guidelines set in 1991 need updating. Based on the latest science, here is a rough idea of what your healthy daily diet should include.

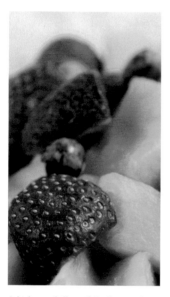

A balanced diet with plenty of fresh fruit and vegetables is a key element of successful running.

Fruit and vegetables

The UK government's recommended daily intake of five portions of fruit and vegetables is not enough for runners. Try to eat two 80g (3oz) portions of fruit and three 120g (4oz) portions of vegetables every day. This may seem similar to the UK guidelines but the portions are larger.

Which vegetables?

You should include vegetables from each of the following five groups in your diet every week:
• Dark green vegetables, such as broccoli, spinach and watercress – three portions a week.
• Orange vegetables, such as carrots, butternut squash, sweet potatoes – two portions a week.
• Beans, lentils, chickpeas – three portions a week.
• Starchy vegetables, such as potatoes – three portions a week.
• Other vegetables, such as cucumber, tomatoes and cauliflower – six portions a week.

Lots of colours

By eating a colourful variety of fruit and vegetables, you will be able to enjoy a healthy selection of vitamins and minerals in your diet. Broccoli and bananas, for example, provide the potassium that is essential to balance the fluid levels in your body, while sweet potatoes are packed with vitamin A to maintain healthy digestion.

Dairy

The calcium in dairy foods ensures that we have healthy bones, while the high protein content helps to repair tissue damage after a run. Aim to eat three portions of low-fat or fat-free dairy products every day. A portion could be a 300ml (10fl oz) serving of skimmed milk, two small pots of yoghurt, or 40g (1$^1/_2$oz) cheese. Vegans can chose calcium-fortified fruit juices or soya milk. Foods containing probiotics, such as yoghurts and fermented dairy products, promise to improve wellbeing by boosting healthy bacteria in your gut. They have also been shown to shorten a cold by as much as two days.

Fat

You should get roughly 25 per cent of your daily calories from fat, but keep your intake of saturated fat to less than 10 per cent, and avoid transfats (see page 67) altogether. Aim to include six teaspoons of oil in a 2,000kcal diet. Half an avocado or 25g (1oz) nuts counts as three teaspoons. Always read the label, and avoid processed foods that include the word 'hydrogenated' in the ingredients list.

Grains

Grains can be divided into two subgroups: whole and refined. Try to make at least half the grains you eat whole grains. For a 2,000kcal diet, aim to eat six portions daily. One slice of bread, one small bowl of

must know

Personal pyramid
Work out your personal food pyramid, based on your age, sex and the amount of exercise you do, by logging on to: www.mypyramid.gov

Go ahead and reward yourself with a treat after a tough race.

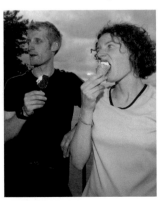

cereal and 25g (1oz) of (dry) pasta, rice or oats all count as one portion. The unrefined versions of bread, rice, pasta and porridge will provide you with slow-release energy, and the high-fibre content will keep you feeling full and satisfied for longer, making a guilty grab for a chocolate bar far less likely.

Meat and beans

The foods in this group are a great source of protein but they can be high in fat, so limit your intake to about 150g (5oz) daily as part of a 2,000kcal diet. One portion equals: 25g (1oz) lean meat, fish or poultry, one egg, one tablespoon of peanut butter, or two tablespoons cooked beans or lentils.

Treats

Since it's an American invention, the food pyramid even takes into account your need for a treat every now and then. If your daily diet includes 2,000kcals, roughly 250 of these are discretionary, meaning you can use them how you like. For instance, you might want to eat more of one of the above groups, or treat yourself to a bar of chocolate. A 300ml (1/2 pint) glass of beer is 200kcals, a glass of wine is about 100kcals whereas a Mars Bar is 230kcals. Don't use running as an excuse to indulge any more than this.

Healthy snacks
Good fats, such as Omega-3, will help to speed up recovery and give your immune system a boost. If you are looking for a healthy snack between meals, a handful of nuts is hard to beat. They're high in protein and unsaturated fat – the healthy kind – that the body slowly converts to energy.

Iron deficiency

Iron is used by your body to create oxygen-carrying red blood cells. Consume enough iron and your aerobic performance may improve, but fail to get the recommended daily amount and you may become anaemic – watch out for headaches, fatigue and above-normal breathlessness during training.

Sources of iron

Try to eat at least three portions of iron-rich food every day. Red meat, seafood, poultry, nuts, beans and eggs are all great sources. You can improve your body's ability to absorb iron by as much as three times by consuming some vitamin C at the same time. Try a glass of orange juice with your fortified cereal in the morning, or add some sliced fresh orange to a spinach or watercress salad.

Make sure you include colourful fruit and vegetables in your diet as well as whole grains, protein and dairy products.

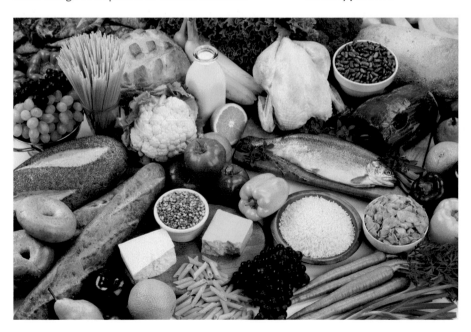

Other diets

Certain diets may present pitfalls for runners, but, with a little care, your running will not suffer. Here are some of the more common diets and how they can affect your performance.

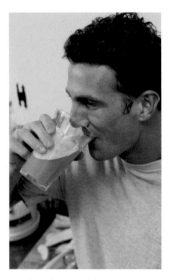

The vitamin C in a glass of orange juice will help you to absorb iron next time you have iron-rich food.

The vegetarian runner

It is possible to perform at the highest level on a vegetarian diet, but training hard does require a good supply of protein for muscle regeneration, so it's important to include adequate amounts of high-quality protein in your diet. Protein is also essential for creating the red blood cells that transport oxygen around your body when you run, and to give your immune system a healthy boost.

Steak out

It's a myth that the best-quality protein comes from red meat. The most readily available source of complete protein, i.e. protein that contains all the essential amino acids, is actually soya. Other plant proteins are incomplete, so it is a very good idea to combine foods that complement each other.

You should try to eat at least two of the following foods at every meal: grains; nuts and seeds; soya products; and pulses. Unless you are a vegan, dairy products and eggs also provide good-quality protein even when they are eaten alone.

Top up vitamins and minerals

Vegetarians will also need to take particular care to consume enough iron, zinc and vitamins D and B12. Pumpkin seeds and pecans provide zinc, while soya products and yeast extract are packed with vitamin B12. To top up your vitamin D levels, be sure to spend some time outdoors every day – the UV hitting your skin will create vitamin D – or you can try eating vitamin D-fortified cereals, yoghurts and spreads. Green, leafy vegetables, such as broccoli, watercress and kale, are a great source of iron.

Ditching the dairy too

Vitamin B12 is essential in red blood cell production and the more you run, the more you need, but it is mostly found in animal products, so vegans need to pay particular attention to including it in their diets. Yeast extract spreads, such as Marmite, as well as fermented soya products will give you a boost but if you're worried you might not be getting enough, take a supplement. Vegan diets can also be low in calcium, so aim to include calcium-rich vegetables, such as spinach and broccoli, as well as sesame seeds, almonds and brazil nuts in your diet.

Diabetic diets

If you have type-1 diabetes and are dependent on insulin, running can help to improve your sensitivity to insulin and improve your blood glucose levels, as well as giving you all the healthy benefits of regular exercise. You should always aim to eat a low-GI carbohydrate snack an hour before you run to provide you with enough slow-release energy to maintain your blood sugar levels. Make sure that the snack includes some bread, potatoes, pasta, rice, or cereals, since the body converts the starch in these foods into sugar to supply the energy that you will need.

want to know more?

- Look out for new varieties of fruit and vegetables to make your daily diet colourful and nutritious.
- Check out some cookery books for healthy, tasty recipes.
- Pick up a healthy eating guide in your local supermarket, or visit www.tesco.com for a free personalized diet profile.
- Visit the Vegetarian Society website at: www.vegsoc.org
- Visit the Vegan Society website at: www.vegansociety.com
- Visit the Diabetes UK website by logging on at: www.diabetes.org.uk

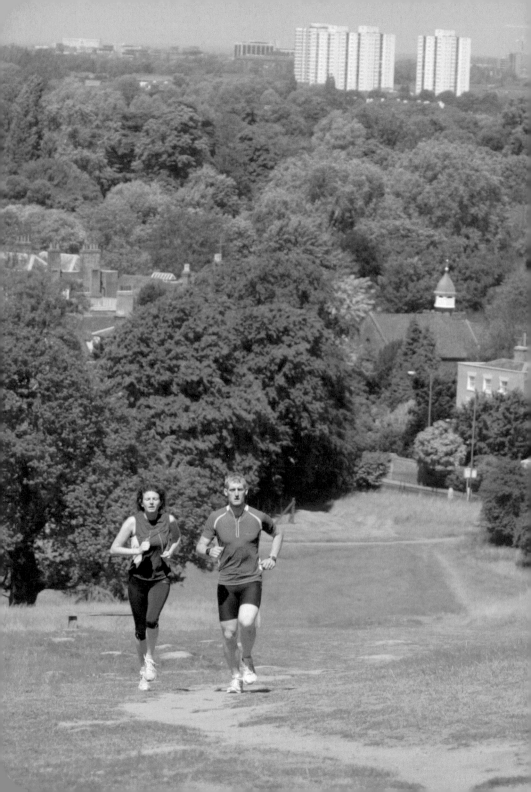

4 Motivation

Even the most dedicated runner needs a little extra inspiration every now and then. There will always be those times when life seems to stand between you and your workout, but with a little creativity, running will become as natural as eating breakfast or taking the dog for a walk. So when there don't seem to be enough hours in the day or you're coming up with new excuses not to run, just flick through this chapter and motivation will never be a problem again.

Making time to run

Running is a simple sport. You can do it on your own almost anywhere at any time of day. The pressure of time ruins more running programmes than knee or foot pain, but it doesn't have to. You can squeeze regular runs into your life, and these time-saving strategies will ensure that you never skip another run.

must know

Missing a session
Even committed runners struggle to do every run they plan. If you miss a session because you have to work late, or there's an emergency, treat it as a blip rather than a crisis. Any successful running programme has to be flexible. Don't try to make up the lost run; just forget about it and resume your programme where you left off. Make running fit into your life rather than fitting your life around running.

Book it

Treat your run as you would any other appointment in your diary – book the time and the date in advance. These then become non-negotiable chunks of time for you to run. Better still, recruit colleagues to join you on a run and you'll be less likely to fail to keep that appointment with your running shoes.

Short but sweet

It's tempting to think distance is everything when you're new to running but you can have a great workout in 20 minutes by throwing some speed play into the session. Tempo runs, intervals and fartlek provide a high-quality session in a short time.

Rise and shine

Getting up half an hour earlier two or three times a week will give you more time to run. Plan ahead: lay out your running kit before you go to bed and put it far enough away that you have to get out of bed to reach it. When the alarm goes off, slip into your kit, have a cup of coffee or a sports drink, head out of the door and start running. You will be surprised how good it feels throughout the day knowing that you have already run.

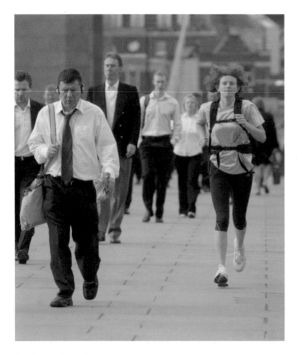

Miss the bus

Instead of jumping in the car or on the train for your daily commute, run some or all of the way to or from work. Running to work is better than running home if you have changing and showering facilities at your work place. Commuting on foot is one of those rare win-win situations. You will save money and create time to run out of what is otherwise dead time.

Working lunch

Don't trail round the shops during your lunch hour; use this time to run instead. If there are no showers at work, start and finish your run at the local gym, or spend 20 minutes on the treadmill. You might be surprised to find out that midday exercise will make you more alert and productive in the afternoon.

must know

Lunchtime runs
Why not encourage some of your work colleagues to join you on a lunchtime run? It's a great way to motivate each other and take a healthy break from your working day. Pick some days of the week when you are going to run and try to stick to them; that way you will develop a routine that others can join in with.

Staying motivated

There are hundreds of reasons to run, and, equally, hundreds of excuses to miss a training session. If you are tempted to miss a run, just remember the following points to stay motivated, and running will soon become a regular part of your life.

must know

Boost your metabolism
If you need a reason to run, remember that not only will you burn calories during your workout, but you'll burn them afterwards, too. That's because running raises your body's metabolism - the rate at which you burn calories - enabling you to shed the pounds more easily.

It's good for you

Running will have a positive impact on your health. It protects against heart disease, depression and many kinds of cancer as well as reducing stress and giving you more energy. In fact, it is one of the best preventative medicines you will find. In addition, running burns fat faster than any other form of aerobic exercise, it's good for your skin, and it will help you look and feel younger, too.

Losing weight

Running is the best calorie-burning workout around, which is great news if you are trying to lose weight or to maintain your ideal weight. You will burn about 100 calories for every mile you cover and you are also more likely to eat a healthier diet when you exercise regularly. Combine the two and you have every dietician's recipe for successful weight loss. Remember that you need to create a calorie deficit if you want to lose weight. By burning more calories than you consume every day, your body will be forced to use stored fat for fuel. The result? You lose weight.

Don't be self-conscious

It is hard not to be self-conscious when you start running. You wonder if everyone is staring at you;

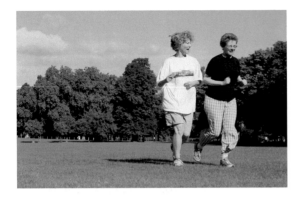

Find several regular training partners with whom you can run on different length or paced runs.

or if you are running 'correctly'. It's unlikely that you are being watched, but if you are worried you should find an environment where other people are running or exercising, such as a park or the gym, and you will feel less conspicuous. It won't be long before running gives you the confidence to run where you like and when you like.

Striking a deal

There will be times when you really don't feel like running, but instead of missing your run altogether make a deal with yourself that you will go out for just 10 minutes. The chances are that once you are out there and into your stride, you will want to carry on past the 10-minute mark.

Sweet dreams

You will sleep better if you follow a regular running programme, which is great news if you are one of the thousands of adults in the UK who are currently sleep-deprived. Sleep deprivation has been linked to depression, poor concentration and even to obesity. Run well and sleep well and you will be a happier and more focused person.

must know

Short but sweet
Even if you only have 10 or 20 minutes to spare for a run, a little is always better than nothing at all. And if you're new to running, going out for a short run is actually better for your body than running for an hour at a time just once or twice a week.

Entering a race

If your running needs a focus, you could sign up for a race. Once you're committed to running a certain distance, on a certain date, you will have a compelling reason to stick with the training and not to give up.

Take small steps

Don't compare yourself to other runners when you are starting out. It does not matter whether you are fast or slow, whether you can run a mile or a marathon, or whether you come first or last in a race. What matters is that you're taking your first running steps. Celebrate your achievements, enjoy the fresh air and surround yourself with people who will support your new passion and might even share some of the running with you. Whether you run with your partner, kids, friends, colleagues, club mates or even the dog, you're less likely to skip a run if you know that you will be sharing the miles.

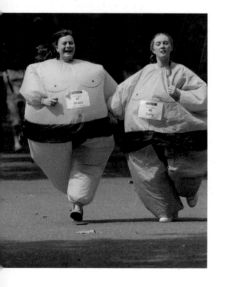

Run in fancy dress with a friend and you're sure to have fun.

Money matters

Involving a charity in your new passion will raise your commitment to your training. Once you know that your chosen charity – and your sponsors – is counting on you, you are less likely to miss a run. As further motivation, you could bet a friend that you can stick to your schedule or reach a particular goal: research suggests that you're more likely to hit a target if there's money riding on it.

Setting realistic goals

If your goal is so tough that achieving it might take you years, you will soon lose interest. Try instead to set yourself short-term incremental goals. For instance, you might give yourself two months to lose 3kg (7lb), say, or plan to run your first 10K. Keep your training interesting by varying your routes, your training partners, and the pace at which you run.

You'll feel good

You might have heard some people talking about a 'runner's high' that they experience after a workout. It is easy to become addicted to that feeling of satisfaction when you have just completed a tough session. If your motivation is suffering, just remind yourself how great you'll feel after the run.

You'll save time

Feeling that you are much too busy to fit in a run can really dampen your motivation, so next time that you have too many demands on your time, why not just remind yourself that running is one of the most time-efficient ways in which you can exercise. After all, you can do it anywhere at any time without having to get in the car and drive to the gym or head for a football pitch. Just pull on your running shoes and head out of the door for an instant workout.

must know

Check out the competition
Running will provide you with endless opportunities to flaunt your competitive streak. You might not even realize you had one until you step across the start line of your first race and begin to plan how you will complete the distance in the quickest time possible. Whether you are racing against the clock, friends or other runners, a little healthy competition is a great way to stay motivated.

By entering a race you can give your training a real focus.

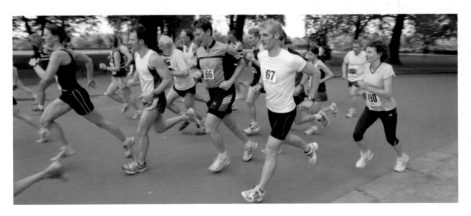

The most common excuses

You may feel a blister coming on or ignore the alarm clock when it's time to get up for a run. The excuses not to run are endless, but so are the benefits when you do exercise. Here are the most common excuses for not running, with advice on how to beat them.

I don't have time

It's a cliché but if you want something done, ask a busy person. The busier you are, the more you can cram into your day. You can make the time for running by going out first thing in the morning, commuting on foot, or by going out at lunchtime. Once you realize the positive benefits it will bring to your life, running will soon become one of the first things that goes into your diary.

I'm not fit enough

You don't need to be fit to start running – if you can run for a minute then you're ready. Run for a minute, then walk for a minute. Repeat it until you can do it comfortably 10 times, then start playing with the run/walk ratios. Try to extend the running sections without increasing the walks.

I'm not built for it

You might not have the whippet-like physique of a Kenyan marathon runner, but you can still run – it's in your DNA. That does not mean, however, that you will be able to run fast or far, but everyone has the physical tools to run. In any case, you will be surprised how quickly regular running can change your physique.

It hurts

If your legs and lungs are burning on every run, then you are running too fast. Slow down. It is normal for your legs to ache the day after a run – after all, you are asking your leg muscles to do something they are not used to doing. The stiffness indicates that your damaged muscles are recovering, and when they stop aching they will be a little stronger than they were before.

People will laugh at me

You might feel self-conscious the first time you step outside to run – children might make a joke at your expense, or you might get whistled at. Don't let this put you off if it happens to you. Remember that you are taking the first steps to a healthy, new you. Before long you'll be crossing the finish line of your first race, and then you will know how good it feels to be part of the running community.

must know

A four-legged friend
Countless studies show that people who own dogs take more exercise than their sedentary counterparts. Your dog's enthusiasm for the great outdoors is sure to force you out of the door in the morning, and once you're out you can enjoy the run together.

You can run anywhere at any time. Create opportunities for running, such as while your kids are busy playing football.

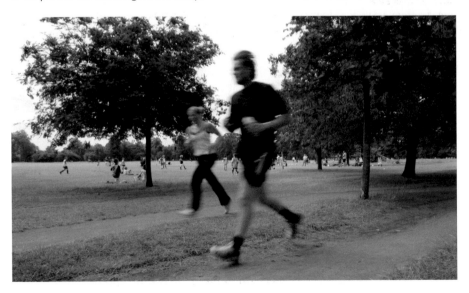

must know

Reap the reward
Instead of making
excuses not to run, try
to create reasons to
train. If you need an
extra incentive, reward
yourself when you stick
to your weekly schedule.
Knowing that a treat,
such as a new pair of
running shoes or a
massage, will be your
reward can make the
difference between
staying in bed or getting
out and running.

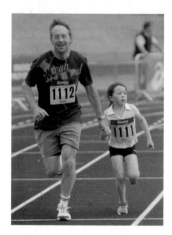

Try to involve your family in your
new hobby. Many races offer fun
runs that the whole family can
enter. They're a great way to
introduce children to the sport.

It's boring

Running, like any other aspect of your life, can
become boring if you cover the same ground every
day, so try to vary your routes together with the
surfaces you run on. Train with different people.
Run on the treadmill at the gym while you catch
up on the day's news. Running can be as interesting
as you want to make it.

It'll damage my knees and joints

Running is a natural activity for which our bodies
are designed. Research carried out on long-term
runners shows that they have stronger joints and
ligaments than non-runners, and they also have
a lower incidence of osteoarthritis in later life.

I don't have the discipline

Sticking to a new running regime can defeat some
people. Ask yourself why you want to run. When
you know what your goal is, you will find it much
easier to complete a programme. Find out what
works for you. For some people, running with a
regular training partner is enough motivation to
ensure they never miss a run.

I won't have time for my family

It is perfectly possible to spend time with your
family and run – you just need to be creative.
Take the family to the park: you can run while your
children accompany you on bikes. Run laps around
the pitch while they are playing football, rugby or
hockey. If your children are a little older, encourage
them to join in, then enter some events that
include junior events or a family fun run.

It's too hot/cold/wet to run

'There's no such thing as bad weather, just bad kit.'
This is an old Russian saying and it's true. With the
quality of lightweight, modern running kit, there is
no reason to be uncomfortable on a run ever again.
If it's raining, then grab a lightweight waterproof.
If it's cold, pull on a pair of running tights, a warm
jacket and a hat and some gloves to protect your
extremities. When the sun is beating down, a hat
and shades will keep you looking and feeling cool.
And if you don't have the kit, try running on the
treadmill at your local gym.

**Running through some inspiring
landscapes will help to keep the
sport fresh and fun.**

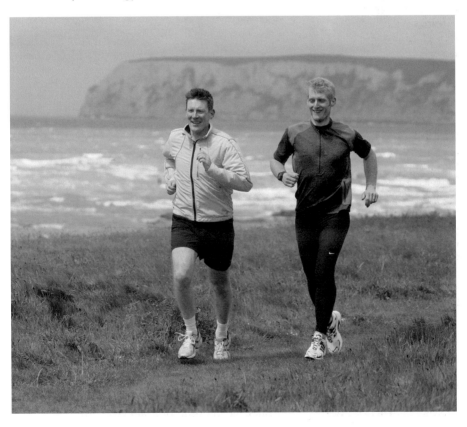

Goal setting

If you need a reason to run, you should have a goal in mind each time you set out. This might be to run all the way around the block without stopping. While you are running, imagine how the training you are doing will help you to achieve your goal.

Set yourself targets

Write down your goals on post-it notes and then display them in a prominent place to provide a constant reminder of your target. If you want to lose weight, list your motivations on a piece of paper and then stick it to the fridge. As you start to see results from your efforts, you will be inspired to carry on. You already know that your goal should be SMART – specific, measurable, achievable, realistic and timed – but just how do you reach it? Having fun is the key. Have you ever noticed how much easier it is to get things done when you are enjoying yourself?

By making running enjoyable you are more likely to reach your goal and have a great time along the way. There are hundreds of ways in which you can make a run more enjoyable – chat to friends, listen to your favourite music, explore somewhere new, enter a race, or mix your running up with another activity, such as cycling.

Take aim

If you feel flat and directionless after achieving a goal, give yourself time to celebrate your achievement and then set yourself a new target. For example, if you've run a marathon, you might want to take a month off before you start thinking about your next goal.

Solo or sociable?

Sometimes running alone is good – in the silence you can listen to your body and be alone with your thoughts – but for many runners it is easier to stick to a schedule and find motivation if they run with a training partner or as part of a group.

Finding a training partner

Start by finding a running partner who has a similar goal to you. If you are both new to running you can enter your first race together, or if one of you has a little more experience, encourage each other to set new personal bests. Running with a friend on a regular basis is the single best way to stick with a training programme because you know you will be letting your friend down if you miss a run.

However, you do not have to limit yourself to a single training partner. You can run with different people depending on what you're trying to achieve on a run. When you're doing a long, slow session, for example, don't run with someone you usually

must know

Chatting
When you're on a long run with a friend or club mates, chatting is a great way to gauge whether you're running too fast. If you're out of breath and struggle to keep a conversation going, then you are running too fast.

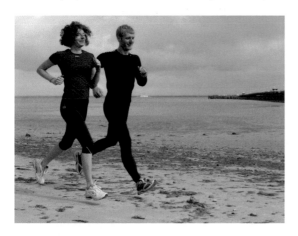

Running with a friend is a great way to stay motivated, but be sure to vary your routes, too. Try running somewhere new in order to keep things fresh.

must know

Online interaction
Running can be a lonely sport, and many runners like it that way, but if you want more social interaction, try going online. The internet offers a variety of opportunities to interact with other runners. You could start a blog (web log) about your training or visit a running forum where you can ask other runners about anything from the best pre-race breakfast to how to train for a marathon.

compete with – you will end up pushing each other to run faster than you should.

If you are doing a tempo run, however, ask someone who is a little quicker than you to set the pace. Keeping up with them will force you to put in more effort than you might if you were running on your own, and while you're struggling for breath they might even offer words of encouragement.

A performance aid

You will find that running with your friends, family, colleagues or club mates helps the miles pass more quickly and more enjoyably, but if you are still not convinced, there is evidence to suggest that training with a partner will also improve your performance. Running clubs have realized that training in a group is a great performance aid. Many runners find it easier to run tough intervals in a group and head to their clubs for regular speed training sessions.

Running to music

If you cannot train with a partner, then why not team up with some music instead? It's hard not to pick up the pace in an interval session when Freddie Mercury belts out 'Don't stop me now', and if you are facing a long run alone, music can distract you and help you relax. It might even make you brighter too: research suggests that running with music improves your cognitive performance.

The safety issue

A word of warning, however: clamping headphones to your ears when you are running outside can cocoon you from noises such as cars, bicycles or

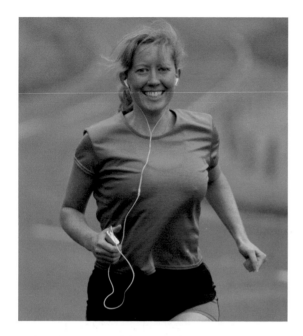

Choose your favourite tunes as the soundtrack to your next run.

pedestrians approaching you. Think about leaving the headphones at home unless you are in a safe environment or on the treadmill.

Audio books

Listening to music while you run has been popular for years but now audio books are adding another option to load onto your MP3 player. There are thousands of books to choose from in book stores and record shops, or you can try the internet.

Book clubs

Why not multi-task by setting up a running 'book club'? You can discuss the book you've been reading with your fellow runners on your weekly long run and engage your brain while forgetting about the miles going by.

want to know more?

• Find inspiration in others' success: *Running Made Easy* (Lisa Jackson and Susie Whalley) features real runners' success stories.
• Mix up your running with another sport. Adventure racing often includes mountain biking and kayaking, or try a triathlon. See Chapter 7.
• Take a running holiday. Meeting other runners has a positive impact on your running. Visit: www.209events.com and www.sportstours.co.uk
• Women looking for running partners should check out the Women's Running Network, which has groups around the country. www.womensrunning network.co.uk
• Commit to a charity event; your motivation levels will soar. Check: www.runnersworld.co. uk/charity

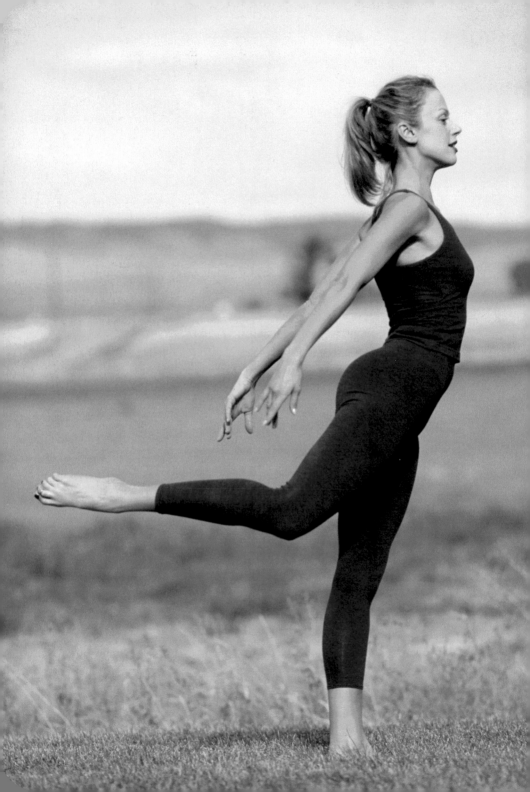

5 The healthy runner

It's estimated that 70 per cent of runners will develop injuries every year. Fortunately, most of these injuries are self-inflicted and can be prevented with a little common sense and a better understanding of your body and how it works. However, injuries are not the only health issue facing runners. Coughs, colds and other minor ailments can all derail your running. Here's how to start healthy and stay that way.

Listen to your body

Running and injury seem to go hand in hand, but you can avoid becoming one of the statistics by listening to your body and making sure that you never increase the speed, intensity or distance of your runs by more than 10 per cent in any week.

must know

Take it slowly
The single easiest way to avoid injury is to increase your mileage gradually. It's easy to forget this when you are new to running and want to pull on your running shoes every day, but by alternating your running days with rest or cross-training days, you will reduce your risk of injury and enjoy the benefits of a variety of workouts.

Dealing with aches and pains

When you're new to running, many of the aches and pains you feel are simply an indication that your body is becoming stronger as it adapts to the new demands placed on it. These aches and stiffness are caused by delayed onset muscle soreness (DOMS) and will generally improve after 48 hours. If pain persists longer than a couple of days, you may have damaged something and you should continue resting. If it's still painful to run after a week, visit your GP for professional advice. On page 112 there are details of other health care professionals who will be able to help with diagnosis and rehabilitation.

A healthy immune system

Maintaining a healthy immune system will cut your risk of illness and infection. A varied diet and staying hydrated enable your body to recover from injury, fight off viruses and give you energy to train. There's evidence to suggest that moderate exercise boosts your immune system, but after a long run or a bout of particularly intense exercise, it may be weakened. Counteract this with a sports drink that contains carbohydrate during exercise: it stabilizes blood sugar and lowers the amount of the stress hormone cortisol that is released during prolonged exercise.

You can also give your immune system a boost by eating certain foods. Vitamin C is a great source of antioxidants, which protect against the free radical damage caused when you exercise. You probably already know that oranges and other citrus fruits are packed with vitamin C, but kiwi fruit and dark berries are also a great source. Defence cells, which attack any invading bacteria when your immune system is weak, are given a boost by vitamin B6, which is found in chickpeas, carrots and bananas. Garlic – and other vegetables from the onion family – contains allicin, which has antiviral properties. You can also boost the good bacteria in your gut by eating leeks and artichokes, which are a good source of probiotics.

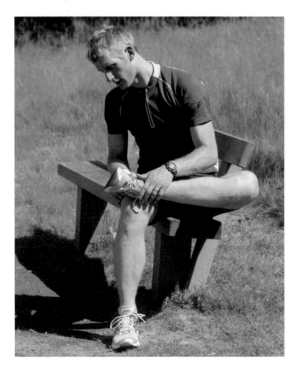

Running in worn-out shoes can lead to injury. Check your shoes regularly and replace them if they are nearing the end of their useful life.

Common running injuries

Your legs and feet take the strain of every running step and are consequently the most common site for running injuries. The chances are that if you get injured, it will be one of the following six problems. Here's how to identify the problem and treat it and, more importantly, prevent it happening in the first place.

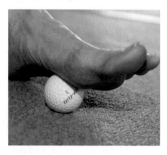

Rolling a golf ball under your foot will stretch your plantar fascia.

Plantar fasciitis

The plantar fascia (a thick band of tissue connecting your heel to the base of your toes) may become torn, inflamed or overstretched when you run. If you feel pain at the base of your heel when you step out of bed in the morning, it's possible you have plantar fasciitis, especially if the pain subsides as you walk around and the muscle warms up, losing its stiffness.

Avoiding it

Plantar fasciitis is often caused by tight Achilles tendons and calf muscles, which should be stretched after every run. High arches or flat feet, as well as wearing old running shoes that do not support your feet may also lead to this injury. Don't be fooled into thinking the injury is improving if it hurts less as you walk around on it – the muscle is simply warming up and becoming less stiff.

Curing it

Rest will help to heal plantar fasciitis, but you can also try this simple exercise: place a golf ball under the arch of your foot and roll it up and down, to the base of each toe and back. Put enough pressure on the ball that you feel a stretch, but not pain.

must know

Ice therapy
As an alternative to the golf ball (above), stretch your plantar fascia and relieve the pain at the same time by rolling a cylindrical block of ice under the arch of your foot. Make the cylinder of ice by freezing water in a paper cup.

If the injury persists, see a podiatrist. They will examine your biomechanics and gait and make footwear recommendations. If overpronation is putting a strain on the plantar fascia, the podiatrist may prescribe orthoses, which are personalized insoles specially designed to correct biomechanical problems. Wear a splint at night to lightly stretch your Achilles tendon and plantar fascia while you sleep, or try acupuncture – new research suggests it can effectively treat plantar fasciitis by targeting points in the arches of the feet and calves.

Achilles pain

The Achilles tendon attaches the middle of the back of your heel to your calf. A sack of fluid, called a bursa, separates it from your heel bone to allow free movement. Place too much stress on the tendon – running uphill is a common cause – and it can become inflamed. The pain usually builds up gradually but can be sudden, and the tendon will feel sore above the heel when pressure is applied.

Avoiding it

You will be susceptible to Achilles pain when you are new to running if you train too intensively and overload the tendon. It can also affect experienced runners when they make a change to their training, such as adding more hill work, speed sessions on the track or wearing some new running shoes.

Curing it

Achilles pain is unpredictable – it may clear up rapidly in a matter of one or two weeks if treated early, or it can take months to treat. To alleviate the

must know

RICE
This is the acronym for rest, ice, compression and elevation. It's an ideal first step for any sprain or strain that leads to inflammation. When you feel pain, the first thing to do is rest. Use ice on the injured area for no more than 20 minutes, at intervals of five hours. Wrap a bandage round the ice pack to hold it in place, taking care not to cut off the blood flow by pulling it too tight. If possible, elevate the injured area above your heart. If the injury doesn't respond in 48 hours, see your doctor.

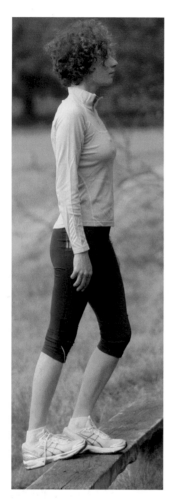

Try this exercise to stretch a tight Achilles tendon.

pain, ice the Achilles and elevate your leg – to prevent any swelling moving down into your foot. Heel lifts in your shoes – of no more than 1cm ($^1/_2$in) – can also relieve pressure on the tendon.

One of the major causes of Achilles pain is a tight calf muscle putting pressure on the tendon. As soon as it is comfortable for you to do so, you should start stretching and strengthening exercises. Try the following exercise to strengthen your Achilles.

Stand on your toes on the edge of a step. Move your body weight to your injured leg and slowly lower your injured heel while keeping your knee straight. Use your uninjured leg to rise up again on your toes. Work up to three sets of 15 repetitions and repeat every day for three months.

Shin splints

Shin splints are a catch-all term for any injury to the muscles, tendons or surface of the bones in your shins. They start with shooting pains up your shins while you're running, but you may also feel pain when you're walking if the injury worsens.

Avoiding them

Shin splints are one of the most common injuries experienced by new runners. They are caused by increasing mileage more rapidly than your body can cope with. Running on hard surfaces, such as roads and pavements, wearing shoes with inadequate cushioning or wearing old shoes will only make the problem worse. Note that shin splints can also be confused with compartment syndrome, which is inflammation of the fascia, the thin covering over your muscle compartments.

Curing them

Shin splints are an overuse injury, so rest, ice and anti-inflammatory drugs will aid recovery. If you overpronate you will be more susceptible to the problem, so check that you are wearing the right running shoes. Stretch the muscles, tendons and nerves in your shins by lying on your back with your right leg in the air. Wrap a towel or belt around the ball of your foot, then pull it with your left hand, bringing your foot down to the left. You should feel a stretch in the outside of your lower leg and ankle. Pull your foot to the right and you'll feel a stretch in your calf. If rest and ice don't improve the injury, visit a physiotherapist.

must know

Instant relief
For immediate relief from shin pain, kneel down with your heels together, toes flat on the ground. Sit back on your feet to create a soothing stretch in your shins.

Try this simple stretch to recover from shin pain.

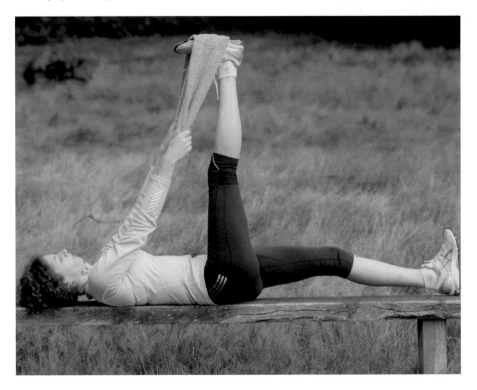

Runner's knee

Pain felt beneath your knee cap when you run
may well indicate that you have runner's knee
(chondromalacia). When you run, your knee cap
needs to move up and down smoothly. If it's not
moving smoothly, it can rub on your femur (the
large bone in your thigh), and irritate the cartilage
that lines the back of the knee cap, causing pain.
The knee cap may appear a little swollen.

Avoiding it

An imbalance in the muscles in your thigh – the
quadriceps – may cause runner's knee. Runners
often have a weak inner quadriceps muscle (your
inner thigh) and stronger outer quadriceps, which
prevents the weaker quads from supporting the
knee cap, with the result that it becomes pulled
or twisted out of place. The knee cap might not
move smoothly due to overpronation, leg-length
discrepancy or iliotibial band tightness. Increasing
your mileage, intensity or changing your running
surface might also lead to runner's knee.

Curing it

Ice your knee for 15 minutes after a run, and take
an anti-inflammatory. You can strengthen your
inner quadriceps by going out cycling. At the gym,
you can use the leg-press machine to strengthen
your inner thighs. You should work one leg at a
time, lowering your leg 30 degrees from the starting
position. Gelatine supplements may also help to
reduce knee pain. If the problem persists, you might
need orthoses to correct an anatomical inefficiency.
If so, seek professional advice.

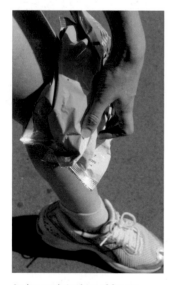

An ice pack (or bag of frozen
peas) can help to relieve
muscular aches and pains.

Iliotibial band (ITB) syndrome

Your ITB extends along the outer thigh from your hip to just below your knee. It stabilizes your knee and absorbs much of the impact of running. If it becomes tight, it may rub against the outside of your knee or hip joint, creating a dull, constant pain while you're running, although it usually stops hurting as soon as you stop running.

Avoiding it

Running on cambered or uneven surfaces may pull your ITB tighter – your leg bends inwards instead of straight forward – and biomechanical issues, such as overpronation or a misaligned pelvis, can also put strain on your ITB. Women have a wider hip/knee angle than men, making them more susceptible.

Curing it

If you feel pain and there is swelling, then take an anti-inflammatory. Three to four weeks' rest and stretching are the usual treatments for persistent ITB pain. Try this stretch: stand with your right leg crossed behind your left and lean to the left, keeping your right foot pressed into the floor; you should feel a stretch along the outside of your leg from your hip to your knee.

Hamstring pain

The hamstring is one of the most common injury areas for runners. A sudden movement can overstretch the muscle and cause a tear or pull, resulting in anything from mild discomfort to eye-watering pain. The area might appear bruised and feel sore to the touch. The repetitive movement of

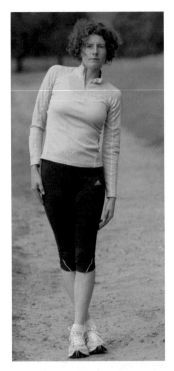

This exercise will stretch your iliotibial band.

must know

Less strain, less pain
Stretch your ITB and ice it every time you run to reduce the pain. If you train on a cambered surface make sure your injured side is higher up – this will place less strain on your ITB.

running can also lead to overuse injuries, which often take longer to heal than tears because you return to running before they've healed properly.

If you feel pain in your hamstring when you're not running, you may have a problem in your back. Pain in the sciatic nerve, which passes down the back of your thigh, is often felt in the hamstring.

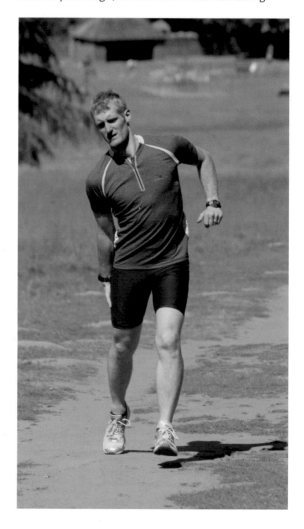

If you feel pain when you are out for a run, stop and stretch the area gently. If there is no improvement, walk home.

Avoiding it

Warm up slowly: it's easy to injure cold muscles with a sudden explosive movement. Don't increase the intensity of your training too quickly as this could lead to an overuse strain – changing your running shoes, altering the surface you run on, or training on a camber can also trigger a strain.

Curing it

After a hamstring injury, regain flexibility before you start to strengthen the muscle. Lying on your stomach, gradually raise one foot until your knee is bent at a 90-degree angle, then lower it. Start with 8–15 repetitions, three times a week. Starting in the same position, repeat the exercise but this time with the raised leg straight. Complete 8–15 repetitions, three times a week.

must know

Support and warmth
To support your hamstring muscle and keep it warm when you run, wear compression shorts or a neoprene sleeve around your leg.

Try this exercise to strengthen an injured hamstring.

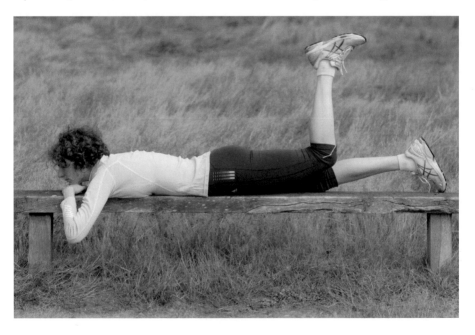

Health care professionals

If you have already tried rest, ice, stretching and strengthening to rehabilitate a running injury with no positive results, then it is time to seek professional help. Here are some of your options. Turn to the back of the book for the websites and contact numbers of all the relevant organizations.

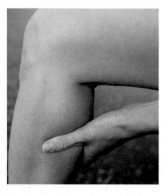

Targeted self-massage can help to relieve inflammation.

Your doctor

The first step into professional medicine should be a visit to your GP. If it's a simple injury, they may be able to treat it; if not, they should be able to refer you to the correct specialist (most private insurance companies insist on this GP-referral before they will cover your treatment costs).

Sports physiotherapy

A physiotherapist is generally the next step (or even sometimes the first step in the private arena). They will actively treat your symptoms and will try to pinpoint the cause. They may examine your gait by watching you run on a treadmill before prescribing specific stretching or strengthening exercises to aid your recovery.

Podiatry

Podiatry is the analysis and treatment of gait and posture inefficiencies. Your feet may be the root of your problem – if they roll in excessively (overpronate) or are flat, for example – but a podiatrist will also look at your whole body. If strengthening exercises cannot balance inefficiencies, they may prescribe custom-made or off-the-peg insoles called orthoses.

Check that they specialize in sports podiatry before making an appointment.

Chiropractic

Many runners will turn to chiropractors when they have back and neck problems. A chiropractor manipulates the bones and joints in your body by applying pressure to realign them.

Osteopathy

Osteopaths also apply pressure to your body but they concentrate on the muscles, tendons and ligaments rather than the bones.

Sports massage

The jury's still out on whether sports massage is effective in treating running injuries, but many runners agree that it relieves tension in muscles and improves circulation and flexibility.

must know

Acupuncture
This is a popular alternative therapy for runners. Fine needles are inserted into the lines of energy in the body to promote healing and relieve tension. Visit the British Acupuncture Council's website (see page 186) to find an accredited therapist.

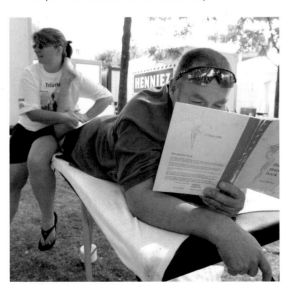

Massages are offered after many events. Why not treat yourself to one after your next race?

Returning to running after injury

Injuries are frustrating. They stop you running, eat away at your hard-earned fitness and are also likely to cause you discomfort and pain. While it is tempting to rush back into training as soon as possible, a gradual return to running is a more sensible option and all part of the general recovery process.

must know

Finding the cause
It's not enough to recover from an injury; you need to pinpoint why you became injured in the first place. Did you increase your mileage or the intensity of your training too sharply? Are your shoes right for your gait? How much time did you spend running on hard roads, or up and down hills? Dealing with the cause is key to preventing the injury reoccurring.

Get real

When you're returning to training after injury, take things slowly. Be realistic about your loss of fitness: it will depend on how fit you were before your injury, how long you've been exercising, and how long you need to rest. If you have a good base level of fitness, you will return from injury more quickly than if you are new to running.

Two for one

A rule of thumb is that it takes about two weeks of retraining to make up for every week of non-running. That means that you lose fitness twice as fast as you gain it, which just goes to show that life is not fair. If you're new to running it may take a little longer to return to your pre-injury fitness levels. Recovery also becomes slower as you age, so if you're 40 or over, be particularly careful during the rehabilitation process.

Over-training after injury

By acknowledging that your fitness levels have declined, and reining in your eagerness to return to pre-injury training intensity, you'll avoid one of the most common running mistakes – over-training after an injury. Pushing your body to work hard at this stage may exacerbate problems because your muscles and tendons may have lost some of the blood vessels that circulate oxygen.

Pool your resources

Cross-training will prevent your blood vessels closing down and minimize your risk of re-injury. Pool running – jogging in deep water while using a flotation belt to keep you upright – is a great way to continue to train while you're injured. Your body is supported by the water and you can still preserve your running fitness.

Take care

Avoid the cycle of re-injury when you resume your running by sticking to a defined schedule. Make sure that you do not increase distance, frequency and intensity – the three key variables in your training – at the same time.

must know

Eat well
When your body is recovering from an injury and you are just beginning to run again, it is very important that it receives the best possible fuel. So make sure that you include plenty of fresh fruit and vegetables in your diet: the vitamins and minerals they contain will help you to recover more quickly.

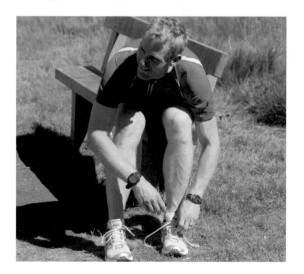

Make sure that you return to running slowly when you are coming back from injury.

Other health problems

Just because you run regularly does not mean that you are invincible. Next time you don't feel 100 per cent, you might find that rest is actually a better remedy than going out for a run.

Should you run with a cold?

When you run regularly, you'll probably feel fitter and healthier than you have in a long time, but you may also find that you pick up more colds. Studies suggest you are vulnerable to viruses or infection when your immune system is weak, which it may be after a long run or a tough race.

You can give your immune system a boost by eating plenty of fresh fruit and vegetables and staying well hydrated. When you have a cold, be particularly wary of running when your symptoms are severe – if you experience a streaming nose, raised temperature or aching muscles. If you only have a blocked nose and a headache, an easy run will probably help.

Osteoporosis

Osteoporosis literally means porous bones. Scientists still are not sure why our bones become weaker as we age, but they have identified ways to promote healthier bones, and running is one of them. In much the same way that your muscles become stronger when you call upon them to work harder, placing demands on your bones when you run forces them to become harder and stronger and thereby reduces the risk of osteoporosis. A diet that is high in calcium (low-fat dairy products, dark green leafy vegetables, tofu and fish) will also help protect bone mass.

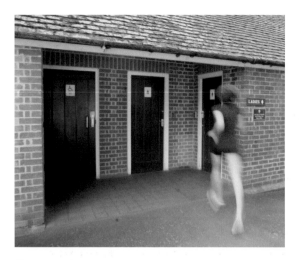

Many runners are forced to take a toilet break when training, but there are steps you can take to minimize the problem.

Runner's trots

This is the catch-all term for a range of symptoms, ranging from cramping and flatulence to nausea and diarrhoea. Runner's trots affects roughly half of all runners during or after exercise. It is likely caused by the motion of running stirring the bowels, or by blood being diverted to the legs and away from the intestine, which triggers cramping and diarrhoea.

Avoiding the trots

If you're regularly forced to make inconvenient pit stops during a run, follow these simple guidelines:
- Start all your runs well hydrated.
- Don't eat for at least two hours before you run: food that is hanging about in your stomach may contribute to the problem.
- Avoid warm fluids and caffeine before you run because they speed up the movement of waste through the intestines.
- Limit your intake of high-fibre foods in the days before a long race.

must know

Be prepared
If you think you might need to visit the toilet before or during a race, it's always a good idea to carry some loo paper in a pocket.

Women's health

Running is a universal sport, where distinctions are made by speed, ability and ambition rather than by sex. Nevertheless, there are some fundamental issues of physiology and biology that impact only on women.

Running and menstruation

Your period can affect how you feel when you go out for a run, but it should not stop you training. In fact, running during your period can actually relieve cramps – as your brain releases feel-good endorphins that reduce the pain – and also alleviate breast tenderness and fluid retention. Do not worry if it feels harder to run in the week before your period: this is the time when the hormone progesterone peaks, making for a higher-than-normal breathing rate. Regular running can also help to reduce the changes in mood that are often associated with premenstrual syndrome.

Amenorrhoea

In some extreme cases, particularly in elite athletes who are on hard training regimes, running can lead to amenorrhoea (the absence of a monthly period). It's due to a lack of oestrogen in your body, caused by over-training, low body fat and inadequate nutrition. The hormone oestrogen is essential for the replacement of bone minerals in your body, and a deficiency raises your risk of stress fractures and osteoporosis. If you start to miss periods – and know you are not pregnant – consider your diet and training levels carefully.

Anaemia

Female runners are at a greater risk of anaemia than sedentary women, due to both menstrual blood loss and the break down of red blood cells when you exercise. This is particularly the case if you're vegetarian. All female runners should aim to consume at least 15mg of iron every day.

Running and pregnancy

Will running damage my unborn baby? Pregnant runners ask themselves this question. The short answer is 'no', particularly if you were a regular runner in good health pre-pregnancy. Although

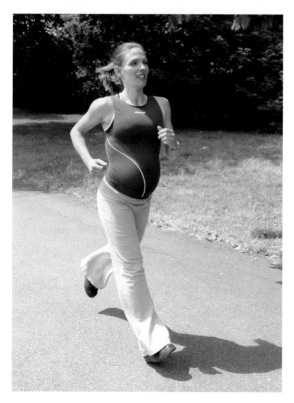

must know

Getting iron
Poultry, fish and lean cuts of beef, pork and lamb will provide a hit of iron. Vegetarians should aim to include fortified cereals, beans, whole grains, green leafy vegetables and dried fruits in their diets. Combining iron-rich foods with foods that contain vitamin C will boost the amount of iron you absorb.

Pregnancy need not mean an end to your running, but you should always seek medical advice before you continue to train.

you should always consult your doctor, there is
no reason why you should not be able to run well
into your pregnancy. Research has shown that
women who exercise during pregnancy suffer less
lower back pain, gain less weight, and have
improved mood and sleep patterns. After giving
birth they're also less likely to suffer from postnatal
depression and will lose weight more rapidly.

Forget the old wives' tale that running can trigger
preterm labour. A study at the University of Carolina
revealed that women who run during the first two
trimesters of their pregnancy are actually 20 per cent
less likely to give birth prematurely than women
who do not exercise vigorously.

Modify your schedule
One potential danger with running during your
pregnancy is a rise in your body temperature. A core
body temperature of no more than 38.3°C (101°F)
could increase the risk of birth defects. To remove
the risk, modify your schedule: forget speed work, hills
and anything that is high intensity. Make sure your
heart beat does not rise above 140 beats per minute.
Drink 100ml (3½fl oz) of fluids once every 15 minutes
to stay hydrated. If it's a particularly hot day, switch
from regular running to pool running: the water will
support you and keep you cool at the same time.

Running post-pregnancy
If you ran regularly during your pregnancy, and
had a normal birth, you could potentially return
to running as soon as a week after giving birth to
your baby. If you had a caesarean section, ask your
doctor when you can return to running. Take it

slowly and try to include plenty of low impact exercises as well, such as swimming and walking. Recent research suggests that running affects neither the content nor volume of breast milk, so breast-feeding should not be a problem, although feeding your baby before you run will make running more comfortable.

Many women are surprised to discover that they can run faster and for longer when they return to running after having a baby. Pregnancy has a similar effect on your body to that of training. For example, when you are pregnant the volume of blood that circulates round your body increases by as much as 30 per cent. This also means that your heart becomes stronger since it has to work harder to keep this extra blood moving. You might also be able to push yourself harder when you run post-pregnancy due to the psychological strength that you have gained from going through labour and the birth of your baby.

Running and the menopause

Very few studies have examined the relationship between running and menopause but those that have suggest that physical activity may help to alleviate menopausal symptoms in some women.

More active menopausal women have reported experiencing fewer mood swings, hot flushes and sweating than sedentary women. However, there is some anecdotal evidence to suggest that women who run regularly may reach menopause sooner. In a *Runner's World* survey, the average menopausal age for runners was 47.6 while the national average was 51 years.

must know

Incontinence
If you're prone to urine leakage, after having a baby the problem can be worse. It's usually caused by weak muscles in the pelvis area which can be strengthened by exercises. In a standing position, contract the muscles in your pelvis as though you were trying to stop the flow of urine. Hold for 10 seconds, then repeat. Try the exercise in other positions, such as sitting or lying down, for five minutes a day. If there's no improvement consult your GP.

Core strength

Good core strength will reduce your risk of injury and also improve your running economy, enabling you to run strongly and smoothly. You'll need to do more than 100 sit ups every morning though. The following moves will help to prevent injury by stabilizing your pelvis and lower spine when you run.

must know

Short circuit
On a day when you don't run, sign up for a circuit training class at your local gym. It's a good cardiovascular workout, and the exercises will help improve your core strength, too.

The exercises

Complete the exercises three times a week. Start off with one set of each exercise and then gradually build up to three. When you attempt these exercises, try to draw your belly button towards your spine.

The gym

The following exercises can be practised anywhere, but if you're in the gym you can also use the equipment there to improve your core strength. Try balancing on a Swiss ball when doing sit ups or press ups, for example. This will engage and strengthen your abdominal muscles to create greater stability and endurance when you run.

Bent knee raise
Lie on your back with your knees bent and feet flat on the floor. Tighten your abdominal wall and slowly lift your left foot 15–30cm (6–12in) off the ground, then lower it. Repeat with the right foot. Lift each foot 10–12 times in total.

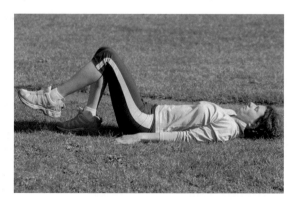

Opposite arm/leg lift

Position yourself on all-fours. Raise your right arm and left leg until they are parallel to the ground and hold for 2 seconds. Return to all-fours, then raise your left arm and right leg. Repeat 8–10 times on each side.

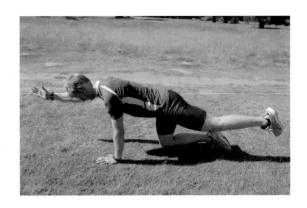

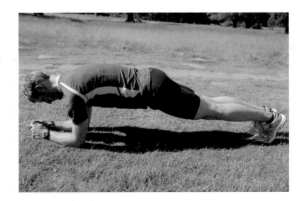

Bridge

Lie on your back with knees bent. Tighten your abdominal wall and raise your pelvis until your body forms a straight line from knees to neck. Hold the position for 10 seconds, then slowly roll back down to the starting position. Repeat 4–6 times.

Plank

Position your elbows shoulder-width apart and directly under your shoulders. Lift your body so it forms a long straight line from your head to your toes. Pull your stomach in and keep your head and neck relaxed. Hold for 20 seconds, then relax and repeat up to 4 times.

Cross-training

This is a great counterbalance to the unique physical demands of running. It will exercise areas of your body that running ignores, give you an active alternative on non-running days and can help maintain your fitness when you're injured. If you are creative with cross-training, your running performance might improve, too.

Types of cross-training

On days when you want to have a break from running, try a non-impact workout, such as cycling or swimming. If the gym beckons, then hop on an elliptical trainer. Set the resistance low so you're not grinding away at a slow pace and aim for a steady cadence on the hills and speed up on the flats. Grip the moving handles for an upper body workout.

Yoga

Yoga is a system of philosophy that originated in India 5,000 years ago. It's a holistic approach to the mind, body and spirit which strengthens and stretches the body through a series of poses, which

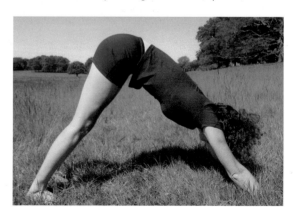

Regular yoga is a great way of gaining more flexibility.

range from low impact to extremely demanding. Yoga is a great way to improve your flexibility if you forget to stretch after every run.

Pilates

This is a series of movements which was originally designed to aid physical ailments and speed up recovery after injury, but it has now been developed into a system for complete body conditioning. Improved core strength is created, using controlled movements and focused breathing.

Pool running

Pool running is a great way to bring your body back to fitness from injury. The water reduces the impact of running by 85 per cent and provides resistance so that your muscles have to work harder to keep you moving. Pool running can also maintain your fitness for as long as six weeks when you are injured.

must know

Pool posture
To achieve the correct posture for pool running, wear a buoyancy belt. This will support your spine and raise your head and chest. Wear an old pair of clean running shoes on your feet, or try AquaRunners, which, along with buoyancy aids, are available from running shops.

Swimming provides a fantastic total-body workout.

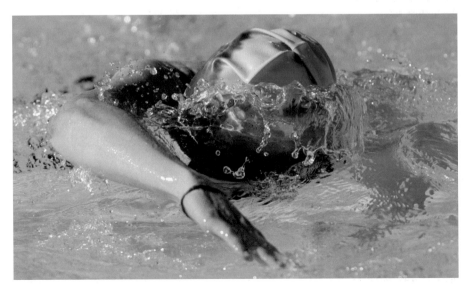

Running safely

You do not just need to protect yourself from injury when you run – you need protection from the external dangers, too. By being more aware of what's going on around you, you will be able to run safely even when you are alone.

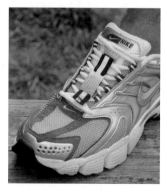

Include your contact details on an ID tag attached to your shoe.

First things first

Before you set out for a run, tell someone where you are going and when you are likely to return. Carry ID, especially if you have a medical condition, as well as a mobile phone or some money for a bus in case you need to stop. You might feel safer if you carry a personal alarm, but you shouldn't rely on it.

The outside world

As you're running, be aware of your surroundings and stay alert to any unusual activities or people. If someone behaves strangely, just turn round and run in the opposite direction. Run towards people and activity, not away from them. Avoid running in quiet areas, particularly during the winter, but if they are the only option, consider running on a treadmill at the gym until the days become longer.

If a car driver asks you for directions, give them from a safe distance instead of approaching the car. If a driver or pedestrian is abusive, ignore them. When there is no pavement, always run facing the oncoming traffic. The *only* exception to this should be on blind bends when you should cross over the road briefly. Don't wear headphones when running anywhere near traffic – the music will make you less aware of what's going on around you.

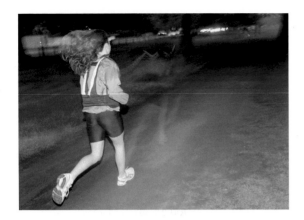

Reflective strips on your kit will help motorists to see you when you are running in the dark.

If you're running in the dark, always wear bright clothes with reflective strips. Protect yourself from changes in the weather by dressing appropriately. In summer, light clothing in technical fabrics will wick sweat away from your body to keep you cool, while a lightweight hat will keep the sun off your head. In winter, several thin layers will help to maintain a comfortable body temperature.

Dog days

It is a dog owner's responsibility to ensure that their pet is always under control but sometimes runners stumble upon a dog that presents a real danger. Next time you're faced with an aggressive dog remember not to become angry, or make lots of noise, as this may antagonise him. Running away may prompt him to chase you, so come to a halt facing the dog, then start to move away keeping a close watch over him but avoiding direct eye contact. If you know you'll be running in an area where there are dogs off their leads, consider carrying a personal alarm. The high-pitched noise may scare a dog and will alert other people that you are in distress.

want to know more?

• Improve your core strength and enjoy a cardiovascular workout at the same time by trying a circuit training class at a local gym. If you'd rather be outdoors try British Military Fitness. Sessions are based on teamwork, motivation and fun and are held in parks throughout the country. www.britmilfit.com
• Ask fellow runners for their injury tips at: www.runnersworld.co.uk/forum
• For up-to-date advice on running health, see: www.netdoctor.com
• Sign up for free sports injury prevention tips at: www.sportsinjurybulletin.com

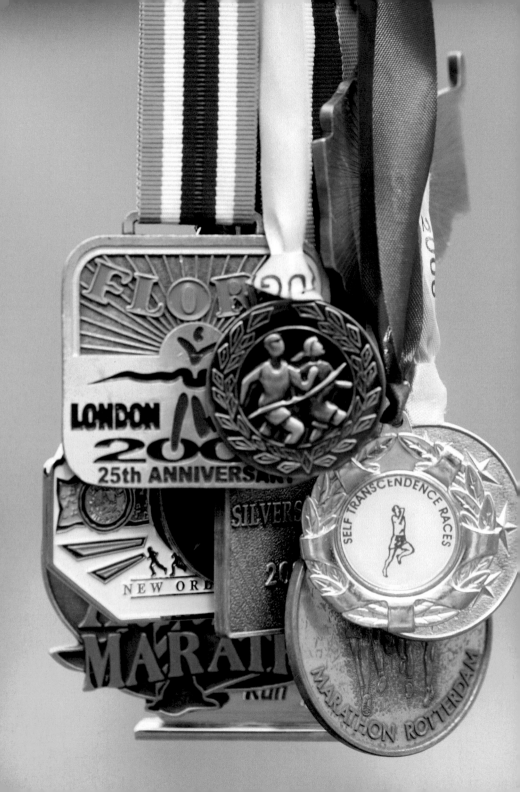

6 Training for racing

Now that you know how to train, what to eat and how to stay healthy, it's time to think about your first race. Don't worry: only a handful of runners are racing to win, for the majority the race is only against themselves and the clock. Nevertheless, races are not only excellent goals to mark your progress but also great fun to participate in. They are infectious, too; once you've taken part in one race, the chances are you will soon be signing up for the next.

Choosing your first race

The high profile of the London Marathon might make you think that it's a good target to aim for. Making your racing debut with a marathon is like tackling Everest after a few weeks of climbing. If you are intent on running 26.2 miles, you should give yourself at least a year to build up a solid endurance base.

must know

Finding a race
There are more than 2,000 races in the UK every year. There's a race search option on the *Runner's World* website (see page 186). Simply key in where you want to run, the month and the distance and a variety of suitable races will appear.

Start with shorter distances

Your first race will be a wonderful, possibly even life-changing, experience but it can also be a little nerve-wracking as you prepare for it. Don't worry if this is the case – it is perfectly natural to be filled with self doubt. Most runners ask themselves: Will I finish last? Will I finish at all? How fast should I run? Am I going to cramp or blister on the way?

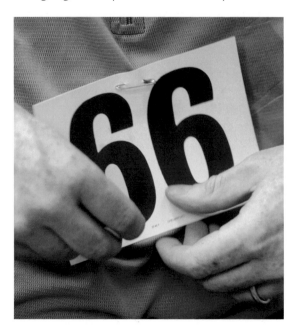

It's a great feeling to pin on the race number for your first race.

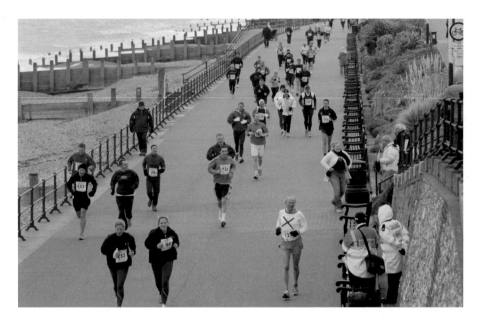

Your first race

Before you start worrying about any of these things, just sign up for a race. Making a commitment to participate is a great way to focus your training by giving you a target to aim for. Choose a race that's close to home to minimize the amount of time you spend travelling. Your friends and family are also more likely to support you if the race is local. Avoid anything that is described as hilly or undulating and look for an event with more than a few hundred runners. The bigger the event, the more likely it is to have a range of running abilities in the field.

Start with a distance you know you can manage. If you are new to running, a 5K is a great place to start. It's challenging but short enough that you can be sure you will finish easily, which will give you confidence for the next race, whether it's something longer or another 5K at a slightly faster pace.

Choose a big event close to home for your racing debut.

must know

Your first race
Sign up for your first race with a friend or someone you've met through your running club. Sharing the experience will make it less intimidating, and you'll have someone to celebrate with when you finish the race.

How to survive your first race

Once you have chosen a race and have started to train using the schedules laid out in Chapter 8, you will need to prepare a strategy to tackle any obstacles that you may encounter before, during or after your racing debut.

must know

Be upbeat
Start the race feeling upbeat and you will be more likely to reach your goal. Research has shown that when you begin a race in a positive frame of mind, you're more likely to stay that way and finish the race more easily than if you allow yourself to become negative.

Do your homework

Try to avoid any unnecessary anxiety before the race. Find out what you can about the course and the event itself. Make a list of things you need for the race – your number, safety pins, racing kit and shoes, towel, plasters, petroleum jelly, post-race snack – and pack your bag the night before. Arrive at the start of the race with plenty of time to spare. Many races attract hundreds, even thousands, of runners making queues for parking, registration, baggage drop and the toilets inevitable. If time permits, walk the last section of the course so you will know what to expect in the closing stages.

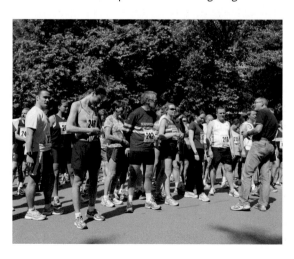

Try to start every race in a positive, relaxed frame of mind.

Cold comfort

If it's a cold day and you have to make your way to the start after dropping your bag, wear an old cotton T-shirt that you can discard when the race begins. Many runners even wear bin liners before a race. This sounds odd but they are a cheap and easy way to stay warm and dry. However, be sure to discard yours responsibly when the gun goes off.

Chips please

If you have chosen to make your racing debut at a large race, try to pick one that issues timing chips to entrants. The advantage of running with a chip is that your official running time starts when you cross the line, not when the gun goes off; at bigger races the difference can be as much as 10 minutes. As a consequence the starts are less frantic and you are more likely to set off at an even pace.

Know your place

Even if the race does not have timing chips, it is worth trying to start in roughly the right place for the time you're aiming for. If you force your way to the front and then set off at a slow jog, you will find yourself in the path of faster runners. It is a similar story if you start too far back: you'll waste time and energy dodging slower runners as you move forward through the field. Many races have a loose seeding, either with roped-off sections or large signs, which try to divide the field by approximate finishing times.

Pace judgement

In your first few races, it is more important that you finish with a smile on your face and bags of

must know

Moving targets
Many runners enter a race with more than one goal in mind. In the first scenario everything is perfect: you stick to your plan, you feel great and you record the time you were hoping for. When things don't go smoothly, it's a good idea to have a 'back-up' goal that you will be happy with, such as equalling a previous best or beating a rival. Even if both goals elude you, don't dwell on your disappointment but consider what went wrong and how you'll emerge a stronger runner.

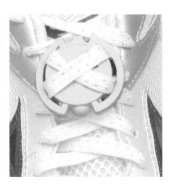

Lace a timing chip into your shoe like this.

must know

T-shirts
If you know there will be crowds of supporters at the race, write your name on your T-shirt. It will make it feel as though everyone has turned out just for you and spectators are much more likely to give you a cheer if they can shout out 'Go on, Alison' than if you are just the anonymous runner in the pink T-shirt.

enthusiasm for your next race than a new personal best. Start slowly and speed up a little in the second half of the race; most novice racers do exactly the opposite. Try not to become obsessed with the time that it takes you to run each mile or kilometre and remember that you're there to enjoy the experience and the atmosphere.

Don't panic

It is perfectly normal for your mood to fluctuate in a race. A bad patch is common, although not inevitable. Instead of becoming demoralized by it, keep going, slowing the pace if you need to, until it passes. If necessary remind yourself of all the tough training sessions you've completed in the build up.

Break it up

It helps if you break the race up into achievable and manageable smaller segments, especially if you are running further than a 10K. Think about the single mile or kilometre in front of you and set yourself a mini target, rather than focusing on all 13 or 26 miles you have to run as a single block, which can feel overwhelming.

Support

If you have identified weak areas in your training, such as the later stages of a distance, ask your friends and family to support you at that point in the race. You will find it hard to give up when you hear them cheering you on. Don't rely on crowd support though if you are taking part in a smaller race where you might find yourself running alone for long sections of the course.

Break through the wall

You've probably heard of runners talking about 'hitting the wall'. It happens in longer races when your body runs out of the readily-available fuel glycogen and has to start burning fat instead, which it can only do at a slower speed. Hitting the wall isn't inevitable though, and it's possible to avoid it if you ensure that your glycogen stores are topped up early on in the race. Do this by consuming anything that contains carbohydrate. You may want to opt for sports drinks and gels, but everyday sweets, such as jelly babies, are just as effective at supplying your body with easy-to-convert sugars to keep your muscles moving. Hitting the wall can be as much a psychological hurdle as a physical one. When you hit a tough patch in the race try not to dwell on how tired you might feel or the blister developing on your foot but instead visualize how great you'll feel crossing the finish line to the cheers of your friends.

Make sure you listen carefully to any pre-race instructions.

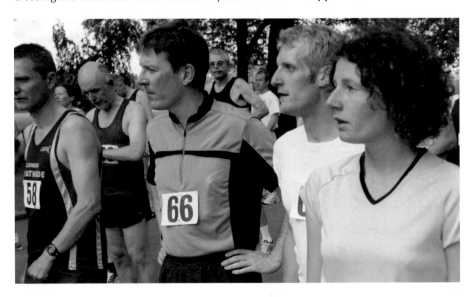

The perfect taper

To ensure that when the big day arrives, you stand on the start line brimming with energy and enthusiasm, you should ease back a little on your training in the run up to a race.

Think about taking a nap the day before a race.

What is tapering?

Traditionally this means reducing the distance you run in the days, or weeks, before a race by 50 per cent, and decreasing the frequency by about 20 per cent, which means cutting down from five to four runs a week. The longer the race, the longer the taper, so if you're preparing for a marathon, you should start cutting back in the two or three weeks leading up to the race, while for a 5K you just need a few days of easier running before you compete.

Less is more

Some runners find that tapering presents more of a challenge than the race itself. After following a schedule and committing to the running it's hard to cut back and put your feet up. Remember that there is little you can do to improve your fitness in the days leading up to a race but there are plenty of things that can go wrong.

Train your brain

The training prepares your body physically for the challenge ahead, but you also need to prepare for it mentally. Visualization is one popular technique you can try. Start by imagining yourself crossing the finish line of the race running strongly. Add as much detail to the image as possible: imagine the kit you

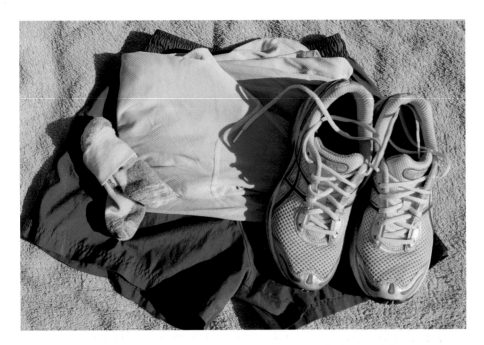

will run in, the sight of your friends waiting to cheer you across the line and the sense of achievement you'll feel as a medal is slipped over your head. You can also try to visualize how you will feel at certain points in the race. Imagine yourself running tall and strong with every step as you run towards the finish.

Before you pack for a race away from home, ensure you have tried out the kit you intend to run in.

Be prepared

Use the time when you're tapering to plan your kit for race day. Wear a variety of kit on your training runs so you have a selection of clothes that you know are comfortable to run in. If you're taking part in a local race, you can choose what to wear when you have checked out the weather forecast, but if you're running away from home, pack a selection of kit so you'll be able to respond to unpredictable changes in the weather.

The perfect race plan

No matter what distance you are racing, it is very important that you have a plan. For instance, it might be to run at an easy pace so that you enjoy the atmosphere of the race, or it might be to run at 7-minute mile pace for the length of a marathon.

must know

Sports gels
Many races now provide sports drinks containing carbohydrate, but if you don't like the taste of the drink on offer, a simple way to replace carbs is by using energy gels washed down with water. A single sports gel contains about 20g of carbohydrate.

Practice makes perfect

Whatever your strategy for running a race, it is vital that you practise it in training to ensure you can actually do it. Try a few shorter runs at your target race pace; experiment with what you plan to eat and drink during the race; and give your running kit and shoes a dress rehearsal. When you line up on the start line, the only new experience should be taking part in the race.

The night before

Don't worry if pre-race nerves lead to a bad night's sleep the night before the race. It's the night before the night before that is more important and, in fact, research suggests that runners who are deprived of sleep perform just as well as those who sleep normally. If you wake up feeling tired, then grab a cup of coffee; the caffeine may also enhance your performance. In any case, the adrenaline that you produce before and during the race will be more than enough to keep you going.

Meal deal

Decide before the race what you are going to eat and drink, if anything, and stick to the plan. You should not need to eat anything in races up to 10K, but if you are going to be running further than this you should consider topping up your glycogen levels with 30–60g of carbohydrate every hour.

How much you should drink is less clear. Make sure you start the race well hydrated by drinking 500ml (18fl oz) of water or sports drink two hours before you run. During the race itself, your thirst is a good natural guide, telling you when to drink, and obviously the warmer it is the more you need to drink to replenish lost fluid.

You should run every race with your own goal in mind.

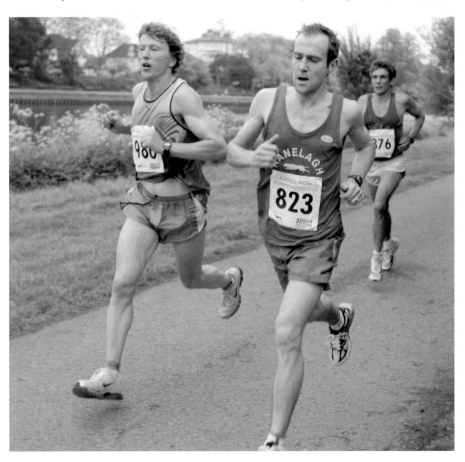

Race tactics

As you become more experienced, you may decide that the time has come to take on your rival from the running club or beat a personal best that has been eluding you. These tactics should help you to perform your best every time you cross the start line.

Try to be negative

One of the easiest mistakes that many new runners make when they feel great at the start of a race is to set off at a pace that is simply too fast for them to sustain. However, a tried and tested way to avoid this is to run a 'negative split', which means that you run the second half of the race slightly faster than the first. Try to hold back in the first half, even if you are feeling good, and start to accelerate from the halfway point onwards.

Catch up slowly

Becoming held up at the start of a race is not a problem if it forces you to start conservatively, but if you need to make up some time you should aim to do this only gradually over the remaining distance. Don't be tempted to speed up so you're back on schedule by mile two, and don't increase your pace by more than 10–15 seconds a mile.

Tuck in close

Professional cyclists draft behind the bike in front and so should you. Look for someone in the field who seems to be running at around your pace or even slightly faster and then tuck in behind them. If the wind is blowing into your face you will be surprised at how much difference it makes running in this way, saving you energy and helping you to run at a steady speed.

Take aim

Set yourself small targets to maintain your focus. Towards the end of the race when you are pushing for the finish, pick a runner who is about 10m in front of you and try to catch them up. Once you are level, pick another runner and repeat the process. Focusing on something other than your tiredness will really help you over a tough final mile.

must know

Personal bests
You'll feel great when you take part in a race and achieve a new personal best. However, instead of easing back and feeling pleased with yourself, this is a great time to sign up for another race of a different distance because the training that you've already put in will translate to other race distances and new personal bests.

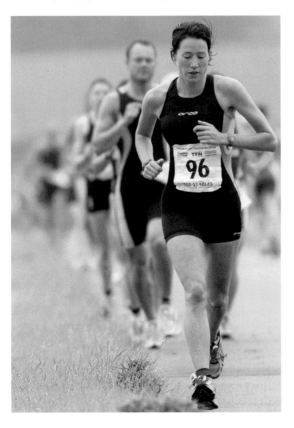

Tuck in behind the runner in front to save energy on a windy day.

Racing equipment

In many sports lightweight, high-tech racing equipment can have a big impact on performance but running isn't one of them. There are some advantages to using specialist racing gear but regular consistent training will reap a greater performance benefit than any equipment. Nevertheless here are some factors to consider.

Shoes first

Racing flats are the stripped-down cousins of your normal training shoes. In an effort to minimize weight, they dispense with most of the normal cushioning and stability features that you would find in trainers. That means you lose the protection, too. If you are heavy (over 11 stone), have any gait problems or expect to run slower than 1:35 for a half-marathon, forget about wearing racing flats.

Light is nice

Although it will not make a significant difference in itself, many runners like the psychological benefit of racing in a lighter shoe. You should try out a performance trainer that is 50–60 grams lighter than a regular trainer but has far more cushioning and support than a racing flat.

Race kit

The same minimalist approach to shoes generally follows for the race kit you wear. For elite men, it's generally a racing singlet, shorts and thin socks; for women, a crop top and briefs. Most ordinary runners prefer to race in well-worn, comfortable training kit. If there is one universal rule for any

must know

SDMs
These can be a useful means of gauging your pace during an event, but the distances on your monitor and the course are likely to be slightly different. The course is measured on the most efficient and direct route a runner can take, but the reality is that only those who are unimpeded at the front can follow it. Don't be surprised if your SDM suggests you're running five per cent further than the race distance.

element of your racing wardrobe, it is never to wear anything for the first time in a race.

Race technology

Increasingly, races give you a timing chip, which clips on to your shoe, to record your start to finish time. Although clocks are usually visible on the course the majority of runners run with a watch both to monitor their time and record their splits every mile or kilometre. Although some like to race with heart rate or speed and distance monitors (SDMs), these are training rather than racing tools.

must know

Socks
These might seem a minor part of your racing kit but they're all that stand between you and a blister. A recent study in the US revealed that avoiding 100 per cent cotton socks is the key to having blister-free feet. Researchers found that nylon socks caused fewer blisters than cotton ones.

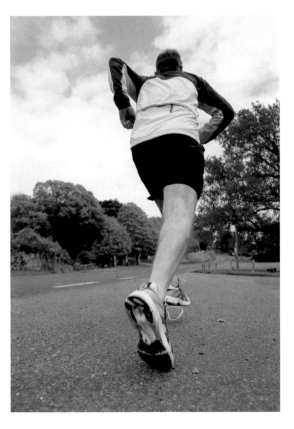

Lightweight shoes such as these might help you to run faster, but save them for races.

Training with a heart rate monitor

Measuring your running in miles and minutes is fine when you are starting out, but if you want to become fitter, faster and stronger, then training with a heart rate monitor will allow you to gauge the true effort you are putting in to every run.

Find your MHR

There is more precision with heart rate monitor training because it is personal to you and how your body is feeling on any particular day. The first step to training using heart rate zones is to find your maximum heart rate (MHR).

MHR formula

For a rough estimate, use the following formula:
- Men: 214 - (0.8 x age)
- Women: 209 - (0.9 x age)

So a 33-year-old woman, for example, would be: 209 - (0.9 x 33) = 179.3.

Treadmill test

To calculate your maximum heart rate more accurately – since some people's can deviate from this estimate by as much as 24 beats per minute – do this simple treadmill test.

Wearing a heart rate monitor, warm up slowly for about 10 minutes, before running as fast as you can evenly for three minutes. Get your breath back by jogging for a few minutes, then again run as fast as you can evenly for three minutes. Note your maximum heart rate (this might be halfway through the three-minute bursts rather than at the end).

Resting heart rate

That's the hard part over – the next step you must take is to measure your resting heart rate (RHR). For the next five days, take your pulse when you wake up every morning. Add the rates together and divide by five to find an average.

Working heart rate

The final step is to calculate what your working heart rate (WHR) should be when you are running. Using the following formula you can calculate your working heart rate at different levels of effort. If you want an easy run at 60 per cent effort, for example, the formula would be:

(MHR-RHR) x 0.60 (per cent effort) + RHR = WHR
So if you have a MHR of 190 and RHR of 55, then your WHR should be 136 beats per minute:
(190 - 55) x 0.60 + 55 = 136

Heart rate zones are roughly divided into:
• Easy (60-75 per cent)
• Moderate (75-85 per cent)
• Hard (85-95 per cent)
These percentages refer to your WHR calculated using the formula above rather than a simple percentage of your MHR.

Monitoring your running

As you become fitter, running a certain distance at a certain heart rate should become easier. On a set route, run at a steady pace and note your time and heart rate. Try the same route again in a couple of weeks at the same steady pace. Your heart rate should be lower on the second run.

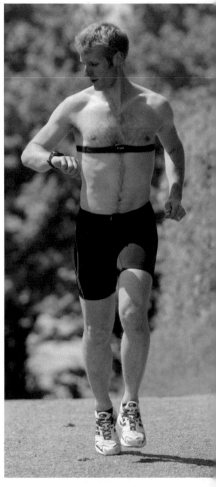

You can use a heart rate monitor to assess your training effort.

Progressing to the next level

You start off jogging a few times a week to improve your fitness or lose a little weight and before you know it running becomes a habit that takes up a big part of your life. Different people will take different things from it, but if you have decided to run more seriously, here's how to progress to the next level.

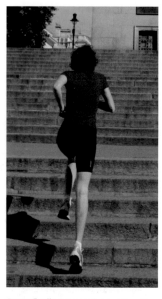

From finding a coach to attending a training camp, there are various steps you can take to progress your running to the next level.

Regularity and distance

Running more regularly should be your first goal when you decide to commit more time to running. If you're currently training three times a week, run an extra day for a month or more before adding runs five and six.

After several weeks of consistent training, your next step will be to increase your overall mileage, probably by starting to extend one of the runs. Build this up gradually by increasing your mileage no more than 10 per cent a week. You can also start to extend the length of some of your shorter runs to about half the distance of your longest run.

Type of training

Once you have developed a strong endurance base, it's time to increase the number and type of speed sessions you run. Try adding some hill work two or three days after intervals. Compared to regular interval training, running hills lowers your injury risk because, even though you're putting in the same hard effort, you're not moving at the same high speed as you do during interval training. Even if you are only running four days a week try to make two of those days quality speed and hill sessions.

Twice as nice

When you're running six times a week and you are including interval training and hill repetitions in your training programme, you may want to consider running twice a day. This is an easy way to raise your overall mileage while protecting yourself from injury. You can even continue to raise the intensity of your training. Two six-mile runs every day, for example, are better than one 12-mile run because you can run each shorter session at a higher pace with less injury risk.

Elite methods

Running further and faster are just two of the ways to take your running to the next level. Here are some of the other methods that many elite athletes employ to become stronger runners.

Find a coach

A coach can create a pathway to a goal that you might not be able to find on your own. He or she will provide you with impartial analysis and motivation and structure your training in a way that allows you to build towards a goal. Whether you recruit the help of a coach from your running club on a formal basis or simply find a more experienced runner to provide you with constructive feedback, the support and expertise will help you to progress.

Camp it up

Another way to focus and receive feedback on your running is to attend a training camp. Again, this can be a formal arrangement at one of the increasing number of weekend or week-long camps, where

must know

Training camps
There are myriad training camps in the UK and abroad. If you want marathon training, Trailplus runs weekend courses, but for a more general approach, try a training camp run by 209 Events (see page 186). Former London-Marathon winner Mike Gratton and his team run training camps in Switzerland, Cyprus, Portugal and Lanzarote. Most of the camps culminate with a race so you have something to train towards during the week you're there.

you will receive the expert advice of professional coaches as well as the chance to train with other runners who are just like you.

Courses and camps are now available on every aspect of running, from technique to training for a marathon and how to tackle the fells. You can also try the more informal approach of taking a week's holiday away with a few running friends to focus on your running.

Taking an afternoon nap could make you a better runner.

Sleep easy

You have probably heard that Paula Radcliffe, the current women's marathon world record holder, takes a two-hour nap every afternoon when she's training. Why does she do this? Well, when you fall asleep, the pineal gland just below the brain releases a natural growth hormone which aids recovery from hard training. Sleeping twice in a 24-hour period will give you two doses of this muscle-building hormone every day.

Prevent injuries first

Nothing messes up a running programme more than getting an injury. If you are increasing the volume and the intensity of your running, you should be aware that you are also increasing your risk of becoming injured.

You should try to change your mind-set about medical professionals, whether they are osteopaths, chiropractors or masseurs, and visit them regularly to treat the injury before you even notice that it has occurred. You may not be aware of them but your body will constantly give out tell-tale signals of any impending problems.

A word on weight

Weight loss can be a confusing issue. Many people take up running to lose weight or keep their weight under control, and your weight will certainly have an impact on how well you perform. Be very wary of linking your performance too closely to your weight, though: healthy weight loss can very quickly switch to unhealthy weight loss if it is pushed too far. It is possible to eat too little and to become obsessed with what you are eating as you might think that this will help you to lose weight and run more quickly. However, being underweight leads to many health problems, so remember that if you are running regularly you are more likely to eat more healthily, both of which will help to control your weight. However, it's still important that you are consuming enough calories to fuel every run.

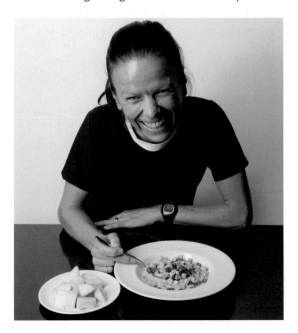

Make sure that you are eating enough healthy calories to fuel your training.

Overdoing it

To become a faster and stronger runner, you will have to train harder. As you start to reap the rewards of that training there is a temptation to train even harder still, but there is a fine line between training hard and overtraining.

must know

Run off-road
Clocking up miles on hard roads and paths can contribute to overtraining injuries. Every time you strike the ground when you are running, oxygen-carrying red blood cells are destroyed. The higher impact forces of hard roads or pavements increase the rate of destruction. Try to run as many of your miles on softer off-road trails and footpaths.

The warning signs

One simple way to find out if you are overdoing it is to get into the habit of taking your pulse as soon as you wake up in the morning. A spike in your pulse rate at any point is an indication of a problem and a sign that you need to give yourself more rest.

More aches and pains
A raised heart rate could also be an indication of imminent illness, which could be linked to a depressed immune system weakened by a heavy

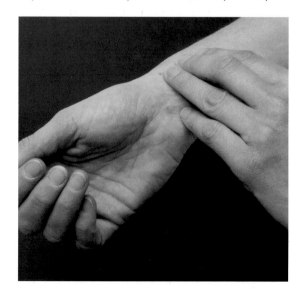

Monitoring your pulse, especially first thing in the morning, will help you to spot the signs of overtraining.

training load. Injuries, particularly overuse injuries like shin splints, are another natural mechanism your body has for telling you that you are doing too much. Finally, think about your motivation – do you struggle to leave the house or come up with more excuses for not running?

Cycle training

Although a schedule is generally a positive element of goal setting and planning, you should not be a slave to it. A good schedule should offer a three to four week cycle of progression followed by a one- to two-week period of relative rest to allow your body time to recover and adapt to the progress.

Junk miles

You may think that jogging for a few miles on a day that should be a 'rest' day is OK but even a short run will prevent your body recovering fully. When it says rest day in your schedule, do just that.

Take off

Don't wait until you are completely exhausted before you decide to take a day off running. You don't even have to cut your mileage; just run a little further on the days when you are scheduled to run and don't run at all on your rest days.

Rest assured

If you think that you might be overtraining, then take a few days off. Drink plenty of fluids, sleep a little longer and reassess your schedule and how realistic it might be. Think about adding more cross-training to your programme for variety.

want to know more?

• For a running holiday with a difference, More Than Just Running has launched the Provence Experience. You will run through vineyards and olive groves before relaxing in farmhouse accommodation. Visit www.morethanjust running.com
• Take your running to the next level by signing up for a running break. The Running Inn in Eastbourne caters for all levels. Log on to: www.therunninginn.com
• Trips to half-marathons, marathons, triathlons and ultras around the world are offered by Sports Tours International www.sportstours.co.uk
• Take a break running round the Queen's back garden in Balmoral with: www.runningthehigh lands.com

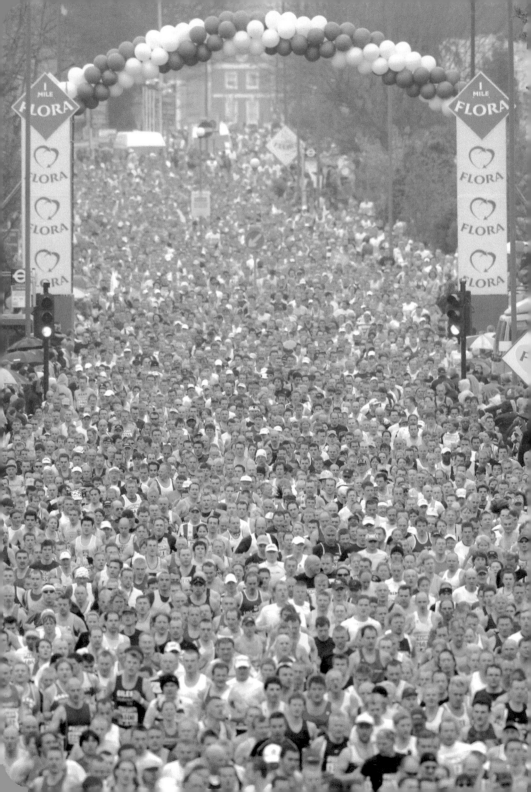

7 What's next?

You are ready for the next challenge but with so many ways to take your running to the next level, deciding what to try next can be confusing, especially when running can take you anywhere in the world. Whether you want to experience running a classic urban marathon, try a tough triathlon, or sign up for a challenging multi-day stage race in a remote corner of the world, there are lots of amazing races out there to test you, and some of these exciting opportunities are featured in the following pages.

Running a marathon

Sooner or later, most runners think about tackling a marathon. It's a huge challenge but one you can comfortably achieve if you have the commitment. Whether you train on three runs a week or six, stick to a schedule and you will cross the finish line.

must know

Marathon origins
The marathon was born in ancient Greece in 490 BC when Pheidippedes ran from the battlefield at the town of Marathon to Athens to deliver news of the Greek army's defeat of the Persians. Legend has it that the soldier spoke one word *niki* (victory), then collapsed and died. The marathon was revived in 1896 when the first modern Olympics were held in Athens. The distance was changed to 26 miles 385 yards at the London Olympics in 1908 because King Edward VII wanted the race to start by Windsor Castle and finish by the royal box in the Olympic Stadium.

Marathons for beginners

Running a marathon has changed dramatically since former Olympic champion Chris Brasher organized the first London Marathon in 1981 when just over 6,000 runners crossed the finish line. The distance has not changed – you still have to cover 26 miles and 385 yards – but back then club runners made up the majority of competitors, while today more beginners are rising to the challenge. There's never been a better time to attempt your first marathon. There are more races to choose from than ever before and more support and advice to spur you towards your goal.

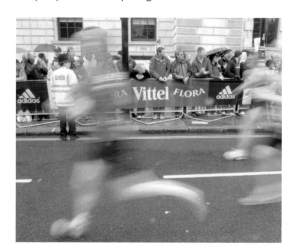

Marathons are great occasions for runners and spectators alike.

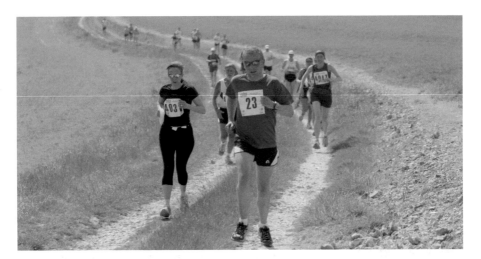

Training for marathons

If you are new to running, build up to the marathon with a minimum of six months' training. If you are already running 30 miles or more every week on a regular basis, you can build up to the marathon distance in about three months.

You can choose from around 50 marathons in the UK every year. They are not all run on roads.

Choosing a marathon

There's plenty of variety on offer. You can choose to make your marathon debut at a big city marathon, such as London or Edinburgh, a rural classic, such as the Loch Ness Marathon, or a more low-key race, like the Kent Coastal Marathon. If your aspirations lie further afield, going abroad to run a marathon can be a truly memorable experience, and a great way to see a new country. For a calendar of marathons held round the world, visit www.aims-association.org. You're sure to find extra motivation during your training if you know you'll be running a marathon at Victoria Falls or among giant redwood trees at the Avenue of the Giants Marathon in California.

Marathon training essentials

You've decided to run a marathon and have started to follow the schedules in Chapter 8. If you follow these 10 essentials of marathon training, you will arrive at the start line in fine form.

Show commitment

Even if you have been running regularly for several years, training for a marathon is a serious undertaking. It has been said that the marathon has ways of finding you out if you have scrimped on your long runs, for example, or dedicated too little time to training. You should start your marathon training acknowledging that your life will be a little different for the next few months. You will be pouring your energy into training, so try to simplify the rest of your life if possible.

Build gradually

You already know that you should build up your mileage gradually when you start to run, and for a marathon this is even more important. You'll be covering greater distances than you have before and need to give your body time to adapt. Always follow a hard run with an easy day.

Run long

The weekly long run forms the foundation of your marathon training. Even if you have to skip other sessions, this is the one you should make a point of completing. It's important to resist the temptation to be greedy though. You only need to do one long run every week – train more and you will increase the risk of injury.

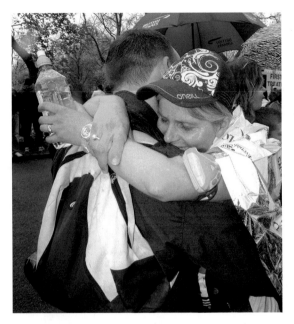

Completing your first marathon will be an emotional experience. Arrange to meet family and friends afterwards to celebrate.

As well as building your endurance, long runs give you the psychological confidence to achieve your goal. Knowing that you can run 20 miles on a lonely training run will help you to breeze through race day when the screaming supporters who appreciate your commitment will encourage your every step.

must know

Shoe shopping
Before you start training for a marathon, make sure you're wearing the correct running shoes. It is also worth buying two pairs, since you will be running more regularly, and covering greater distances. That way, each pair will have a chance to dry out and bounce back before you use it again.

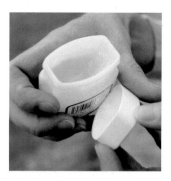

Apply a little petroleum jelly to any vulnerable areas to prevent them chafing when you run.

Live a balanced life

It's not just your training that is important in the build-up to a marathon – your lifestyle will have an impact, too. You might be able to complete a marathon on four hours' sleep a night and a diet of junk food, but you'll find it much easier to recover from the volume of training if your body has a nutritious supply of food and the opportunity to rest well after those long runs.

A successful marathon is as much a mental challenge as a physical one. If there are other major events going on in your life, such as parenthood, a change of job or new house, your training will suffer. Try to simplify rather than complicate your life when you start to train for a marathon and explain to friends and family that you're committed to the training for a finite amount of time.

Dress rehearsal

On your weekly long runs, you can experiment with everything from what you're going to eat and drink during the marathon to what you're going to wear. The marathon is challenging enough without having to worry whether your new socks will cause blisters. You might even want to practise running at the same time of day that the marathon starts.

Do a trial run

If you are aiming at a big city marathon one of the biggest differences you'll notice between training and the race is running in a congested group of runners. You need to practise this just as you practise everything else. Try to run at least one race with a field of more than 5,000 runners in the build-up to your marathon.

must know

Rucksacks
Train with a weighted rucksack if you are electing to run in fancy dress and your costume is heavy. Experiment with your outfit on a long training run: you might discover that it restricts your stride or rubs in certain places and needs adapting.

Ease back

Many runners find that tapering (see page 136) in the last few weeks before the marathon is the most difficult part of their training schedule. During the hard training of the previous weeks you may have been looking forward to the taper, when you can relax a little and don't have to run as far, but it can be torture; you've done the hard training, feel great and simply want race day to arrive. Just remember that other than rest, there is little you can do in the final two weeks to help you run a better marathon, but plenty of things that can ruin it.

Negative splits

After a few weeks of tapering, many runners will fly across the start line of the race, forgetting all their good intentions to start slowly and run a negative split (completing the second half faster than the first). Your pace at the start may feel slow but it's worth holding yourself back – a minute per mile too fast in the early stages of a marathon can cost you five minutes a mile in the latter stages.

Six and out

The last six miles are the true test of the marathon. It's unknown territory for many first-timer runners (long runs often peak at 20 miles) and it's a tough mental battle running with fuel-depleted, tired muscles. This is where everyone suffers, particularly if you started too fast. Try to make sure that you eat some carbohydrate early on in the race, such as some gels or a sports drink, and then try to hold something back for this part of the race, especially if it's your first marathon.

must know

Stitch
Stitches are common running problems caused by cramping in the area of your diaphragm. Start by exhaling hard to clear the air from your abdomen. This stretches the diaphragm muscle where a stitch usually occurs. If that doesn't work, run with your arms raised above your head for a while. It looks silly but this stretches the diaphragm, too.

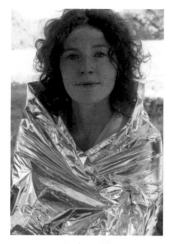

Try to keep warm and dry after a race. Some marathons provide special aluminium foil wraps.

Walk this way

In both your training runs and during the marathon itself, never forget that it's okay to walk. Combining running with walking will improve your endurance because walking eases the fatigue that builds up with continuous running. You can try running for five minutes, then walking for one. In the marathon, walk when you are passing drink or food stations and do it from the first miles onwards.

Fancy dress

Running a marathon is not enough of a challenge for some people – they want to do it in fancy dress. If you decide to become a superhero or dress up as a banana, there are some tips you can follow for a successful costume drama. Fix your name and the name of any charity you're supporting in a prominent position. If your costume restricts access to your mouth or arms, consider how you're going to eat and drink during the race. Ensure your costume won't disintegrate or hold the water if it rains.

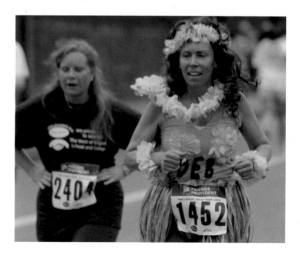

Supporters are sure to give you a big cheer when you wear fancy dress for a race. You may find that your sponsors are more generous, too.

Marathon must-knows

Eat breakfast
Always eat breakfast, even if it means getting up in the early hours to do so. You might not feel like eating but you need to top up your glycogen stores. Aim to eat some porridge, cereal, or bagels two to three hours before the start of the race and make sure you're well hydrated.

Relax at the start
Don't waste energy keeping warm or warming up at the start. Wear something old you can discard in the first mile, and ease into your pace in the first few miles as the field starts to spread out.

Cramp
Cramp is often a result of dehydration. Try to drink little and often during the race, and if cramp sets in, stop and stretch the sore area and keep moving to improve the circulation.

Blisters
Avoid blisters by wearing clean, comfortable socks that fit snugly against your feet and wick away moisture as your feet start to sweat. If you know that you have potential blister hotspots, tape the area or apply some petroleum jelly – to prevent rubbing – before you put your socks on.

Chafing
You can also use petroleum jelly to prevent chafing. These are the points where your skin rubs against itself – between your thighs or under your arms – or where the skin rubs against a piece of clothing. Again, apply a lubricant to suspect areas or tape them. Men often cover their nipples with sticking plaster to prevent chafing.

Ultras

For a small group of runners, the marathon is merely a stepping stone to even longer, harder races. The world of ultra running (events that are longer than a marathon) presents countless racing options, from 30-milers on the South Downs to six-day challenges in the Morrocan Sahara Desert.

must know

Tough events
There are more than 50 ultras held in the UK every year. One of the toughest events is the Marathon of Britain where runners complete 175 miles in six stages on consecutive days. See: www.marathonofbritain.com

Choosing an ultra

Ideally, your first ultra should be flat and in an area that you can travel to easily. You can sign up for an event with testing hills or one that's halfway round the world, when you have a little more experience and have made sure that you enjoy running ultras.

Ultra training

Forget speed and distance when you are training for an ultra – time spent on your feet should be the cornerstone of your running plan. Regular runs of more than three hours are hard on your body, so try to break up the big runs into more manageable blocks spread out over a weekend. Make sure you train on the same terrain that you'll be running on during the ultra. Long, brisk walks can also benefit your preparations, particularly as they come with lower risk of injury. It's also a great mental boost if you know you can walk quickly and maintain a good pace in parts of the race where you might need to slow down to eat or to tackle a hill. Both in your training and racing for an ultra, think of the race in stages, breaking the run up into manageable chunks, rather than starting off worrying about the 50 miles that lie ahead of you.

Adventure racing

If you want to mix your running with some other sports, then adventure racing is a great place for you to start. Events range from individual two-hour 'sprint' races, which involve several different activities, to multi-day team expedition races which require months of careful planning.

Types of events

The events are usually team based (with at least one woman in the team), and they focus on the core disciplines of off-road running, mountain biking and some form of canoeing or kayaking. Like running, adventure races have a designated start and a finish but they rarely follow a set course. Longer races will often require you to have a degree of navigational competence, where picking the best route and trying to follow it is all part of the challenge, whether it's on foot, bike or in a kayak.

must know

What appeals?
Sign up for a UK race that appeals to your sense of adventure on one of these sites:
www.questars.co.uk
www.aceraces.com
www.sleepmonsters.co.uk

Seasonal events

There are more than 1,000 adventure races held worldwide every year, so there are plenty for you to choose from. These range from especially challenging ones that are modelled on the original Raid Gauloises in which racers compete 24 hours a day for up to seven days, to shorter races that you can complete in just a few hours.

The adventure race season takes place in the spring and summer months in the UK, but there are some winter events that are starting to appear on the calendar and if you are prepared to travel there are endless international options.

Spice up your running by mixing it with other sports.

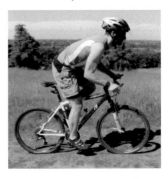

Triathlon

This is one of the fastest growing participation sports in the UK. In the last five years, the number of people who are choosing to swim, bike and then run has tripled and it's estimated that more than 100,000 people will enter a triathlon this year.

Race distances

Many beginner triathletes are actually runners who are looking for a new challenge and have realized that they can combine two of their favourite cross-training workouts with their core activity in a fun multi-sport event. As with running, there are a variety of triathlon race distances from which you can choose, as listed opposite.

Most triathlons start with an open water swim in the sea or a river or lake.

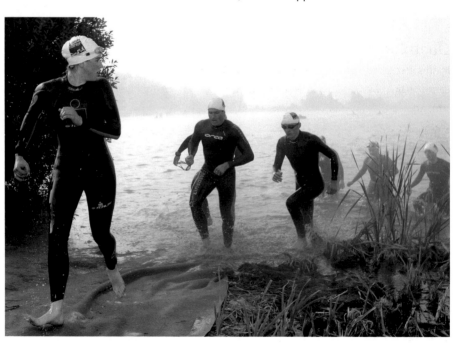

Common triathlon distances (swim/bike/run)
Super sprint – 400m (0.25 mile)/10km
(6.2 miles)/2.5km (1.5 miles)
Sprint – 750m (0.5 mile)/20km (12.4 miles)/
5km (3.1 miles)
Olympic – 1500m (1 mile)/40km (25 miles)/
10km (6.2 miles)
Half Ironman – 1900m (1.2 miles)/90km
(56 miles)/21km (13.1 miles)
Ironman – 3.8km (2.4 miles)/180km (112 miles)/
42km (26.2 miles)

Finding out about triathlon
You can find out more about triathlon as a sport
and even enter your first race by logging on to the
British Triathlon Association's website at:
www.britishtriathlon.org

Duathlon
In this discipline, the races are divided into three
sections but the swim at the start is replaced by a
run, and since you will not need to take a dip in the
water, the duathlon racing season is longer than the
triathlon season. All you will need to take part are a
bike, helmet and a pair of running shoes. Distances
vary, often due to local terrain, from the shorter,
accessible events to the more gruelling races, such
as the aptly named Ballbuster.

A great way to train for a duathlon – which will
also improve your endurance for running – is to
complete a 'brick session'. This means that when
you finish a run, you immediately get on your bike
and go for a ride. It will teach you to carry on when
your legs are tired.

Ten must-do races

Investing time and money in travelling to a race means choosing an event you've always dreamed of running, or one in a destination you want to visit. Here are races that offer something different, ranging from gruelling stage races and marathons in extreme environments to fun runs and relays.

must know

Ask questions
Don't be afraid to contact a race organizer to ask questions before you sign up for a race. Many organizers will be happy to put you in touch with people who have taken part in previous years, so you can get a first-hand account of what's in store for you.

London Marathon, UK

For a big city marathon, London is hard to beat. The course passes some of the capital's most famous landmarks before culminating in a stunning finish outside Buckingham Palace on the Mall. The crowds, atmosphere, camaraderie and the sheer fancy-dress-driven fun of it will stay with you forever. Since the first race in 1981, the London Marathon's popularity shows no sign of waning. Nearly 100,000 people applied for 20,000 public ballot places this year. If you fancy running the London Marathon and want details on how to enter, log on to: www.london-marathon.co.uk

Boston Marathon, USA

The Boston Marathon is the grand daddy of all the big city marathons. The first race took place in 1897, making it the world's oldest annual marathon, and by insisting that only runners who qualify may enter the race it retains a prestige that's absent from many similar events. The course is slightly downhill but it is still considered tough, and to say you have finished the Boston Marathon will earn some serious bragging rights with your running friends. Log on to: www.bostonmarathon.org

Comrades Marathon, South Africa

The world's biggest mass-participation ultra hasn't been around for as long as the Boston Marathon but it has just as much tradition. The 54-mile race was first run from Pietermaritzburg to Durban in 1921 as a tribute to comrades who died in the First World War. South Africa's isolation in more recent times led to Comrades becoming the country's most popular race. The direction the course is run alternates each year. Log on to: www.comrades.com

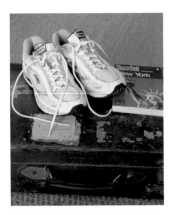

Combine running and travel by entering a race away from home.

Great Ethiopian Run, Ethiopia

You might not think to travel abroad for a 10K, but the Great Ethiopian Run in Addis Ababa is well worth the effort. Look around the start line at many overseas races and you'll notice that competitors

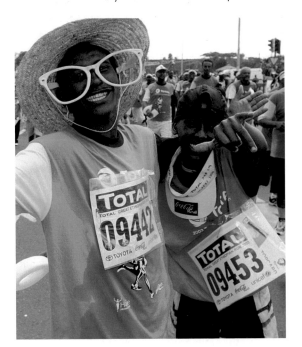

Ethiopia may have produced some of the world's best distance runners, but it also knows how to put on a great 10K.

must know

Dress rehearsal
Practise running in the kit you'll be wearing for the race. You may be taking part in a race that requires you to carry your own kit and food, so prepare yourself by wearing a full rucksack when you run. Find out what food and fluids will be available so you can practise eating and drinking them in training.

are predominantly from Western countries. Here you will be one of very few foreigners, making for a refreshingly different cultural experience.

Don't even think about your time or your place in this race. Addis Ababa is located at altitude and is home to dozens of the world's finest distance runners. If you want to follow in their footsteps, go to www.ethiopiarun.org

Hood to Coast Relay, USA

This annual relay sees teams of between eight and 12 runners tackle the 197-mile course from the slopes of Oregon's Mount Hood to the Pacific Ocean town of Seaside. The race has been going for 25 years and it regularly attracts 12,000 runners. If you don't have a team, the organizers will try to find one for you. To find out more about it, you can log on to: www.hoodtocoast.com

Himalayan 100-mile stage race, India

For a real challenge, head to India for this five-day stage race. The first day includes a climb of more than 5,000ft over 24 miles, although views of four of the world's five highest peaks – Everest, Lhotse, Makalu and Kanchenjunga – will provide a great incentive to reach the finish. The wonderful scenery and tough stages continue for the next four days when you will run from 13 to 30 miles. For more information, look at: www.himalayan.com

Inca Trail Marathon, Peru

At 27.5 miles this is a little further than a marathon but past participants have claimed that it feels more like 50 as you tackle the punishing but beautiful

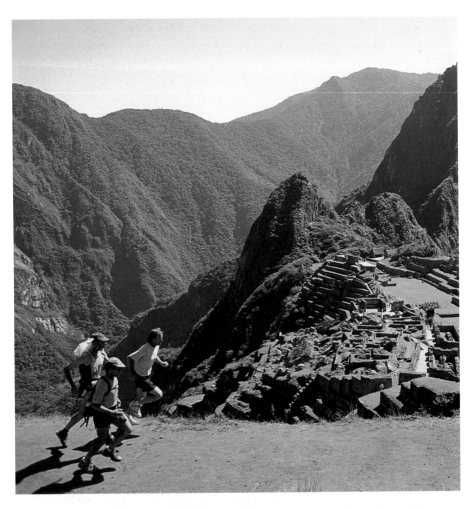

mountain passes of the Inca Trail before arriving at the ancient Inca ruins on top of Machu Picchu. The running may well be tough but the luxurious accommodation and the wonderful sightseeing throughout the rest of the trip will make this feel more like a holiday than a race. If you want to find out more about this amazing race, you can log on to: www.andesadventures.com

You will forget about tired legs with views like this at the Inca Trail Marathon in Peru.

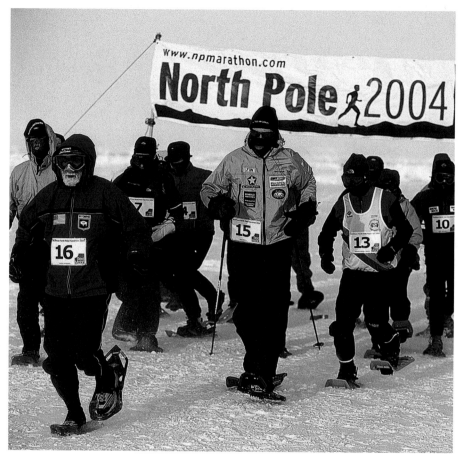

It really is possible to run a race almost anywhere in the world, including the North Pole.

North Pole Marathon

If you want to run where few people have even set foot, head for the North Pole Marathon. Billed as the world's coolest marathon, it takes place at a temporary camp on the ice near 90°N. It's the only certified marathon distance that's run entirely on water – the frozen Arctic Ocean – and is recognized by Guinness World Records as the most northerly marathon on the planet. For more details, see: www.npmarathon.com

Médoc Marathon, France

For something a little closer to home, but no less unusual, the Médoc Marathon near Bordeaux is hard to beat. You should leave your watch at home to truly appreciate the landscape of vineyards and châteaux as you sample local cheese and other delicacies at the 22 food stations. Stop at all 21 wine drinks stations and you might never reach the finish, but if you do, the first and last runners are awarded their weight in wine. Look at: www.marathondumedoc.com

Bay to Breakers, USA

More of a fun run than a serious race, the Bay to Breakers in San Francisco is one giant party of fancy dress costumes from start to finish. As the name suggests, the race starts on the Embarcadero in San Francisco Bay finishing by the Golden Gate Bridge after 12K. More than 70,000 runners take part every year, making this one of the world's biggest, and most memorable, races. Log on to the website at: www.ingbaytobreakers.com

want to know more?

• **The London Triathlon is now biggest in the world. Check out www.thelondontriathlon. com.**
• **You can take your training to the next level by subscribing to a free email bulletin on Peak Performance. Log on to: www.pponline.co.uk**
• **Find out how to qualify for the London Marathon: www.london-marathon. co.uk.**
• **You can search for British races on: www.runnersworld.co. uk/events**

must know

Be prepared
If you're going to be facing unusual running conditions, such as running on sand or snow, in an area of high humidity, or at extreme temperatures, try to simulate the conditions when you train. At the North Pole Marathon, for instance, you'll need to run in snow shoes, so make sure you train in a pair before you go.

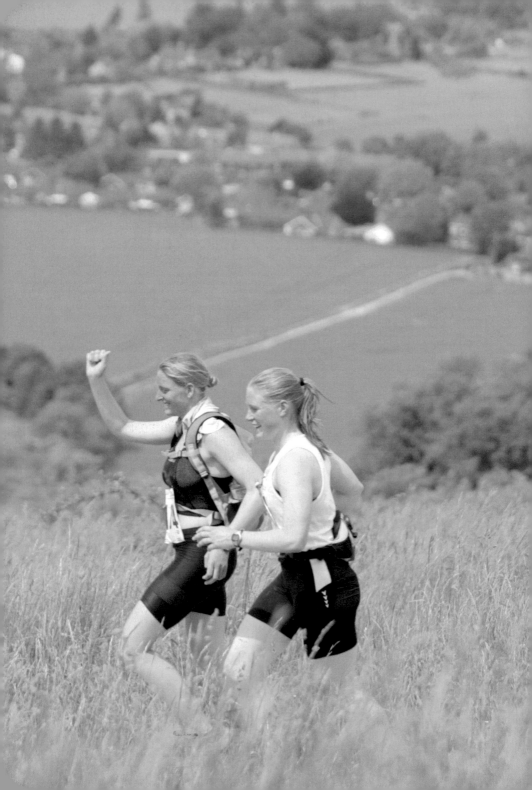

8 Training schedules

Whether you are looking to take part in your first race or want to move up to a longer distance, the schedules featured in this chapter will help to prepare you for any race from a 5K up to a marathon. It is a good idea to start with shorter races, such as 5Ks and 10Ks, to build up your confidence and endurance. Many runners are content to run no further, but if crossing the finish line of a marathon is your ultimate goal, you can find out how to train for it.

Copies of the training schedules in this chapter, and the beginner's programme on pages 26-27, are available to download from: **www.collins.co.uk/running**.

Guidelines

These schedules are made up of sessions that you will already be familiar with. A combination of slow, steady runs, interval sessions, and the all-important rest days, will deliver you to the start of the race in great shape and eager to cross the start line.

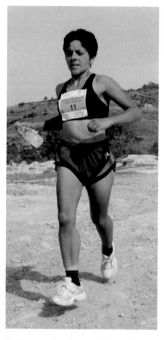

Follow a schedule and you will start every race feeling confident.

Intervals

These fast-paced interval sessions, run at or above the pace you aim to complete a race, will improve your speed and endurance and teach your body to run faster. Faster miles thrown into easy runs help your body cope with changes of pace – something you have to do in a race situation.

Fartlek

The fartlek sessions in these schedules will offer you the flexibility to run hard when you are feeling strong and to choose how long to spend running more slowly to recover. Aim to run harder for at least 50 per cent of the distance you cover in the session, and vary the length of your recoveries. This type of session is good preparation for the type of variable effort that you will encounter in a long run on an undulating course or in a race.

Hill sessions

No hill sessions feature in these schedules, but if you would like to run hills, substitute them for one of the hard midweek sessions, such as intervals or fartlek. Limit your hill sessions to one per week. If there are no hills where you live, try increasing the gradient to more than five per cent if you run on the treadmill. Hill running will build your strength and speed while improving your mental confidence.

Easy runs

Building endurance is the foundation of successful distance running – speed will come afterwards. The easy runs within the schedules are not only designed to condition your body but also to develop the confidence you need to enable you to run as far as the race demands without breaking down. Check that you are not running too quickly by keeping up a conversation with a friend. If you are struggling to gasp out a reply, then you need to slow down.

Rest

A rest day means no running rather than no exercise at all. If you want to exercise on rest days, then try doing a non-weight bearing cross-training exercise, such as swimming or cycling.

DIY schedules

If you would rather have the flexibility to create your own schedule, then make sure that it incorporates the following principles.

- Build up your endurance progressively. For any schedule that lasts more than six weeks, plan your runs in four-week segments and ease back on the fourth week before building again in the fifth.
- Always alternate hard and easy days.
- Most people struggle to stay motivated for any more than three months. If you need longer than this to prepare, say for your first marathon, break your ultimate goal into smaller goals of 6–12 weeks each.
- When you're a beginner, include one hard training session per week; if you are an improver, include two.

5K beginners

If you've successfully completed the run/walk programme on page 24, you're ready to enter your first 5K race. Commit to just three runs a week and in six weeks you will cross the finish line of your first 5K race.

Beginner's 5K schedule

Wk	Mon	Tues	Wed	Thurs	Fri	Sat	Sun
1	Rest	2 miles easy	Rest	2 miles easy	Rest	Rest	3 miles easy
2	Rest	2 miles easy	Rest	2 miles fartlek	Rest	Rest	3 miles easy
3	Rest	3 miles easy	Rest	2 miles fartlek	Rest	Rest	4 miles easy
4	Rest	3 miles easy	Rest	2 miles fartlek	Rest	Rest	4 miles easy
5	Rest	2 miles easy	Rest	3 miles fartlek	Rest	Rest	2 miles easy
6	Rest	2 miles easy	Rest	2 miles easy	Rest	Rest	Run 5K

must know

Be flexible

Few people are able to rigidly stick to a programme. If you do miss a session, don't give yourself a hard time and don't try to play catch-up; just aim to complete the next session on the schedule. If you don't have the time or the energy to complete a whole session, do as much as you can. A little is always preferable to nothing at all.

5K improvers

If you have been running at least three times a week for several months and want to improve your time from a previous race, this schedule should help you reach that goal.

Improver's 5K schedule

Wk	Mon	Tues	Wed	Thurs	Fri	Sat	Sun
1	Rest	3 miles easy	Rest	3 miles fartlek	Rest	Rest	4 miles easy
2	Rest	3 miles easy	Rest	4 miles fartlek	Rest	Rest	5 miles easy
3	Rest	3 miles easy	Rest	1 mile easy, 2 x 1 mile at target race pace, 1 mile easy	Rest	Rest	6 miles easy
4	Rest	3 miles easy	Rest	4 miles fartlek	Rest	Rest	5 miles easy
5	Rest	3 miles easy	Rest	1 mile easy, 2 x 1 mile at target race pace, 1 mile easy	Rest	Rest	4 miles easy
6	Rest	3 miles easy	Rest	1 mile easy, 1 mile target race pace	Rest	Rest	Run 5K

10K beginners

Tackling a 10K race is likely to be the furthest you have ever run. The main aim of your programme is to build enough endurance to run the whole race without stopping to walk. Most of the runs are at an easy pace to develop your endurance, with a few faster fartlek sessions thrown in during the middle four weeks to give you a taste of the faster-paced running. This should also make the longer runs easier.

Beginner's 10K schedule

Wk	Mon	Tues	Wed	Thurs	Fri	Sat	Sun
1	Rest	3 miles easy	Rest	3 miles easy	Rest	Rest	4 miles easy
2	Rest	3 miles easy	Rest	3 miles fartlek	Rest	Rest	5 miles easy
3	Rest	4 miles easy	Rest	4 miles fartlek	Rest	Rest	6 miles easy
4	Rest	4 miles easy	Rest	5 miles fartlek	Rest	Rest	6 miles easy
5	Rest	3 miles easy	Rest	3 miles fartlek	Rest	Rest	4 miles easy
6	Rest	3 miles easy	Rest	3 miles easy	Rest	Rest	Run 10K

must know

Walk first
Try to get into the habit of starting every run with five minutes of brisk walking before easing into the run. Finish with five minutes of walking to cool down and then stretch.

10K improvers

You have probably run a 10K and now you want to improve your time. The emphasis is still on endurance in this improver's schedule, but you will be raising your lactate threshold – the point at which your legs turn to jelly – by completing a mid-week faster-paced session of either intervals or fartlek. Stepping up from three to four days a week requires a significant commitment because you will have to run on consecutive days during the week.

Improver's 10K schedule

Wk	Mon	Tues	Wed	Thurs	Fri	Sat	Sun
1	Rest	3 miles easy	Rest	3 miles fartlek	3 miles easy	Rest	4 miles easy
2	Rest	3 miles easy	Rest	1 mile easy, 2 x 1 mile target race pace, 1 mile easy	3 miles easy	Rest	6 miles easy
3	Rest	4 miles easy	Rest	5 miles fartlek	3 miles easy	Rest	7 miles easy
4	Rest	4 miles easy	Rest	1 mile easy, 3 x 1 mile target race pace, 1 mile easy	3 miles easy	Rest	8 miles easy
5	Rest	3 miles easy	Rest	4 miles fartlek	3 miles easy	Rest	4 miles easy
6	Rest	3 miles easy	Rest	1 mile easy, 1 mile target race pace, 1 mile easy	3 miles easy	Rest	Run 10K

Half-marathon beginners

If you have successfully completed a 10K race and want to move up to a longer distance, the long runs in this 12-week schedule will improve your endurance while the faster fartlek and interval sessions will build your speed endurance. You will find that this schedule includes some weeks when you will complete two hard sessions to prepare you for the challenge of running 13.1 miles on race day.

Beginner's half-marathon schedule

Wk	Mon	Tues	Wed	Thurs	Fri	Sat	Sun
1	Rest	3 miles easy	Rest	4 miles easy	Rest	Rest	5 miles easy
2	Rest	3 miles easy	Rest	4 miles fartlek	Rest	Rest	6 miles easy
3	Rest	4 miles easy	Rest	4 miles fartlek	Rest	Rest	8 miles easy
4	Rest	4 miles easy	Rest	4 miles inc. 2 x 1 mile at target pace	Rest	Rest	10 miles easy
5	Rest	3 miles easy	Rest	3 miles easy	Rest	Rest	6 miles easy
6	Rest	4 miles easy	Rest	4 miles fartlek	Rest	Rest	8 miles easy
7	Rest	4 miles easy	Rest	4 miles inc. 2 x 1 mile at target pace	Rest	Rest	10 miles easy
8	Rest	4 miles easy	Rest	4 miles fartlek	Rest	Rest	12 miles easy
9	Rest	3 miles easy	Rest	3 miles easy	Rest	Rest	8 miles easy
10	Rest	3 miles easy	Rest	4 miles fartlek	Rest	Rest	10 miles easy
11	Rest	3 miles easy	Rest	4 miles inc. 2 x 1 mile at target pace	Rest	Rest	6 miles easy
12	Rest	3 miles easy	Rest	3 miles inc. 3 x 800m at target pace	Rest	Rest	Run half-marathon

Half-marathon improvers

You have regularly run more than 10K in training and racing and now want to compete at the half-marathon distance. The majority of the runs in this 12-week schedule are easy to increase your weekly mileage while limiting your injury risk. Once a week you will complete a hard session of fartlek or intervals. Aim to run the faster efforts at an even pace so be sure to give yourself enough time to recover between faster sections.

Improver's half-marathon schedule

Wk	Mon	Tues	Wed	Thurs	Fri	Sat	Sun
1	Rest	3 miles easy	Rest	4 miles fartlek	3 miles easy	Rest	6 miles easy
2	Rest	3 miles easy	Rest	5 miles fartlek	3 miles easy	Rest	8 miles easy
3	Rest	4 miles easy	Rest	5 miles fartlek	4 miles easy	Rest	10 miles easy
4	Rest	4 miles easy	Rest	1 mile easy, 3 x 1 mile at target pace, 1 mile easy	4 miles easy	Rest	12 miles easy
5	Rest	4 miles easy	Rest	5 miles fartlek	4 miles easy	Rest	8 miles easy
6	Rest	5 miles easy	Rest	1 mile easy, 3 x 1 mile at target pace, 1 mile easy	4 miles easy	Rest	10 miles easy
7	Rest	5 miles easy	Rest	5 miles fartlek	4 miles easy	Rest	12 miles easy
8	Rest	5 miles easy	Rest	4 miles fartlek	4 miles easy	Rest	12 miles easy
9	Rest	3 miles easy	Rest	1 mile easy, 3 x 1 mile at target pace, 1 mile easy	3 miles easy	Rest	10 miles easy
10	Rest	3 miles easy	Rest	5 miles fartlek	3 miles easy	Rest	8 miles easy
11	Rest	3 miles easy	Rest	3 miles fartlek	3 miles easy	Rest	6 miles easy
12	Rest	3 miles easy	Rest	1 mile easy, 1 mile target pace, 1 mile easy	2 miles easy	Rest	Run half-marathon

Marathon beginners

If you have been running more than 10 miles a week for at least six months and want to finish your first marathon, this schedule will help you to cross the finish line without falling apart in the latter stages of the race. Your goal should be to finish feeling strong and able to get out of bed and walk the next day. The emphasis in this three-session-per-week schedule is to build your endurance through the long Sunday runs.

Beginner's marathon schedule

Wk	Mon	Tues	Wed	Thurs	Fri	Sat	Sun
1	Rest	6 miles easy	Rest	4 miles easy	Rest	Rest	8 miles easy
2	Rest	5 miles easy	Rest	3 miles fartlek	Rest	Rest	10 miles easy
3	Rest	4 miles easy	Rest	3 miles fartlek	Rest	Rest	12 miles easy
4	Rest	6 miles easy	Rest	4 miles easy	Rest	Rest	8 miles easy
5	Rest	5 miles easy	Rest	3 miles fartlek	Rest	Rest	10 miles easy
6	Rest	6 miles easy	Rest	3 miles fartlek	Rest	Rest	12 miles easy
7	Rest	5 miles easy	Rest	5 miles easy	Rest	Rest	14 miles easy
8	Rest	4 miles easy	Rest	5 miles easy	Rest	Rest	16 miles easy
9	Rest	6 miles easy	Rest	4 miles easy	Rest	Rest	18 miles easy
10	Rest	5 miles easy	Rest	4 miles fartlek	Rest	Rest	12 miles easy
11	Rest	4 miles easy	Rest	4 miles fartlek	Rest	Rest	14 miles easy
12	Rest	6 miles easy	Rest	5 miles easy	Rest	Rest	8 miles easy
13	Rest	6 miles easy	Rest	4 miles easy	Rest	Rest	10 miles easy
14	Rest	5 miles easy	Rest	3 miles easy	Rest	Rest	Run marathon

Marathon improvers

If you regularly run more than 20 miles a week, and have been running for more than a year, this schedule will help you to achieve your best marathon time yet. The marathon is an endurance event and the foundation of this 14-week schedule is still your Sunday long run. The rest of the time you'll be doing easy runs to enable your body to adapt to your training, and some faster-paced sessions so you can practise your target race pace.

Improver's marathon schedule

Wk	Mon	Tues	Wed	Thurs	Fri	Sat	Sun
1	Rest	7 miles easy	Rest	5 miles fartlek	6 miles easy	Rest	10 miles easy
2	Rest	7 miles easy	Rest	6 miles inc. 2 x 1 mile at half-marathon pace	6 miles easy	Rest	12 miles easy
3	Rest	6 miles easy	Rest	7 miles inc. 4 miles fartlek	6 miles easy	Rest	14 miles easy
4	Rest	6 miles easy	Rest	5 miles easy	5 miles easy	Rest	10 miles easy
5	Rest	5 miles easy	Rest	7 miles inc. 3 x 1 mile at half-marathon pace	7 miles easy	Rest	16 miles easy
6	Rest	6 miles easy	Rest	7 miles inc. 4 miles fartlek	6 miles easy	Rest	18 miles easy
7	Rest	7 miles easy	Rest	7 miles inc. 4 miles fartlek	5 miles easy	Rest	20 miles easy
8	Rest	8 miles easy	Rest	7 miles easy	7 miles easy	Rest	10 miles easy
9	Rest	7 miles easy	Rest	7 miles inc. 3 x 1 mile at half-marathon pace	6 miles easy	Rest	18 miles easy
10	Rest	7 miles easy	Rest	7 miles inc. 4 miles fartlek	5 miles easy	Rest	20 miles easy
11	Rest	8 miles easy	Rest	6 miles inc. 3 x 1 mile at target race pace	6 miles easy	Rest	18 miles easy
12	Rest	8 miles easy	Rest	7 miles easy	7 miles easy	Rest	12 miles easy
13	Rest	6 miles easy	Rest	5 miles inc. 3 x 1 mile at target race pace	5 miles easy	Rest	10 miles easy
14	Rest	3 miles easy	Rest	5 miles inc. 2 x 1200m at race pace	3 miles easy	Rest	Run marathon

Glossary

Adventure racing
A team-based multi-sport event in which the course is usually unknown in advance.

Aerobic
A type of exercise where the muscles use oxygen from the blood as well as fat and carbohydrate to produce energy.

Anaerobic
Exercise where energy is generated from carbohydrates without oxygen.

Biomechanical
The mechanics of the way in which the body moves.

Cool down
The period of time after exercise when you might walk or stretch until your heart rate returns to its pre-exercise level.

Cross-training
Sports and activities that are used to benefit your running, but which are not running, such as swimming, cycling or working out with weights.

Cushioned shoe
Running shoes with a soft midsole and the least added stability.

Duathlon
A race when competitors must run, cycle, then run again without stopping.

Fartlek
A flexible way to do interval training by varying the speed during an extended run.

Footstrike
The contact that your foot makes with the ground when running.

Gait
The motion your foot makes as it comes into contact with the ground.

Gilet
A sleeveless, usually windproof or water-resistant, jacket.

Glycaemic Index (GI)
Method of classifying carbohydrate-rich foods according to how quickly they release glucose into the blood stream.

Glycogen
Carbohydrate stored as fuel in muscles.

Heel counter
Firm material at the back of a shoe that keeps the foot firmly in place and stable.

Hitting the wall
The point when the body runs out of glycogen on a long run or a marathon and has to switch from carbohydrate to fat as its primary fuel source.

Insole
The removable liner inside a shoe that helps with fit and provides your foot with extra cushioning.

Intervals
A set period of fast running repeated a number of times with a short recovery between each effort.

Lactic acid

A by-product of anaerobic exercise that collects in the muscles.

Maximum heart rate

The number of times your heart beats when you're at the peak of physical exertion.

Midsole

The foam cushioning layer on a shoe that sits between the upper and outsole.

Motion control shoe

A type of shoe with features to control severe inward rolling of the foot during the gait cycle.

Negative split

Completing the second half of a race faster than the first.

Outsole

The rubber underside of a shoe that comes into contact with the ground.

Overpronation

Excessive inward rolling of the foot during the gait cycle.

Pose method

A controversial running technique that is supposed to lower the risk of injury and increase the efficiency of your running gait.

Resting heart rate

The number of times your heart beats per minute when you are at rest.

Speed work

A type of training that is specifically designed to make you run faster.

Stability shoe

Shoes that have added support on the inside of the midsole or upper to slow down and limit the excessive inward rolling of the foot.

Taper

The period of time before a race when you reduce your training mileage and intensity.

Tempo run

A run at a hard pace for a sustained period of time. It is also sometimes known as a threshold run.

Trail shoe

A shoe made with a tougher upper and studded rubber outsole to provide more grip on rugged terrain.

Triathlon

A race in which the competitors must swim, cycle and then run a set distance without stopping.

Ultra

A racing distance that is longer than the 26 miles 385 yards of a marathon.

Upper

The part of a running shoe that encloses your foot.

Wicking

The ability of a synthetic fibre to carry sweat away from the body to the outside of the material where it can evaporate.

Working heart rate

Your maximum heart rate minus your resting heart rate.

Need to know more?

There is a wealth of information now available for runners, particularly if you have access to the internet. Listed below are a few of the organizations and resources that you might find useful.

Governing organizations

UK Athletics
Athletics House, Central Boulevard,
Blythe Vally Park, Solihull,
West Midlands B90 8AJ
tel: 0870 998 6800
www.ukathletics.net
The national governing body for UK athletics.

British Triathlon Association
PO Box 25, Loughborough LE11 3WX
tel: 01509 226161
www.britishtriathlon.org
The national governing body for the sports of triathlon and duathlon in Great Britain.

Internet resources

209 Events
www.209events.com
For training camps in Switzerland, Cyprus, Portugal and Lanzarote.

The National Register of Personal Trainers
www.nrpt.co.uk
Find a personal trainer in your area or learn how to become one.

Peak Performance
www.pponline.co.uk
A sports science website for athletes and coaches.

Race for Life
www.raceforlife.org
The UK's biggest women-only fundraising event.

Realbuzz.com
www.realbuzz.com
A running and health website.

Runner's World Magazine
www.runnersworld.co.uk
Online running magazine with free training information and an extensive events calendar. For a comprehensive guide to the races coming up in your area, you can log on to:
www.runnersworld.co.uk/events

Trailplus
www.trailplus.com
Runs weekend running courses.

UK Athletics club and track directory
www.runtrackdir.com
Comprehensive details on the 600 plus running tracks in the UK.

Women's Running Network
www.womensrunningnetwork.co.uk
A women-only network of running groups.

Health websites

AquaRunners
www.mobilishealthcare.com
For buoyancy aids.

British Acupuncture Council
www.acupuncture.org.uk
Log on to find an accredited acupuncturist.

British Chiropractic Association
www.chiropractic-uk.co.uk

Chartered Society of Physiotherapy
www.csp.org.uk
Click on to Physio2u link to find a physiotherapist in your area.

General Osteopathic Council
www.osteopathy.org.uk.

Society of Chiropodists and Podiatrists
www.feetforlife.org
Log on to find a podiatrist.

Sports Massage Association
www.sportsmassage.org
For a national register of sports massage
practitioners.

Running magazines

Athletics Weekly
Descartes Publishing Limited,
83 Park Road,
Peterborough
PE1 2TN
tel: 01733 898440
www.athletics-weekly.com

Runner's World
NatMag Rodale Limited,
33 Broadwick Street,
London
W1F 0DQ
tel: 020 7339 4400
www.runnersworld.co.uk

Running Fitness
Kelsey Publishing Limited,
1st Floor, South Wing, Broadway Court,
Broadway, Peterborough PE1 1RP
tel: 01733 347559
www.runningfitnessmag.com

Fitness magazines

Men's Health
NatMag Rodale Limited, 33 Broadwick Street,
London W1F 0DQ
Tel: 020 7339 4400
www.menshealth.co.uk

Men's Fitness
Dennis Publishing Limited,
30 Cleveland Street, London W1T 4JD
tel: 020 7907 6000
www.mensfitnessmagazine.co.uk

Top Santé
Emap Elan, Endeavour House,
189 Shaftesbury Avenue, London WC2H 8JG
tel: 020 7437 9011

Zest
The National Magazine Company Limited,
33 Broadwick Street, London W1F 0DQ
tel: 020 7339 4400
www.zest.co.uk

Further reading

Books
Bean, Anita, *The Complete Guide to Sports
Nutrition* (A&C Black)
Bingham, John, and Hadfield, Jenny, *Marathon
Running for Mortals* (Rodale)
Higdon, Hal, *Marathon* (Rodale)
Murphy, Sam, *Marathon from Start to Finish*
(A&C Black)
Murphy, Sam, *Run for Life – The Real Woman's
Guide to Running* (Kyle Cathie)
*Runner's World Complete Book of Running for
Beginners* (Rodale)

Runner's World Guide to Running (NatMag Rodale)
Whalley, Susie, and Jackson, Lisa, *Running Made
Easy* (Robson Books)

Audiobooks
To find audiobooks to listen to while you run,
try the following websites:
www.amazon.co.uk
www.audible.co.uk
www.audiobooks.co.uk
www.listen2books.co.uk

Index

Author's acknowledgements

A big thank you to Ant Smith, Cynthia Rowand and Jason Ralph for being
great models, and to Steven Seaton for always finding their best sides.
The weather wasn't perfect but I hope you all enjoyed the shoots as
much as I did. Thanks also to everyone at *Runner's World* magazine for
your support and advice, and for giving me the opportunity to run in
some beautiful - and sometimes dangerous - places.

☼ Collins need to know?

Look out for these recent titles in Collins' practical and accessible need to know? series.

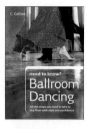 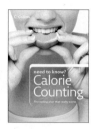 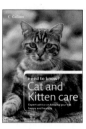 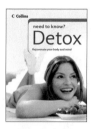 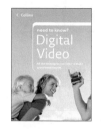

Ballroom Dancing — Calorie Counting — Cat and Kitten care — Detox — Digital Video

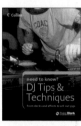 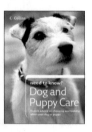 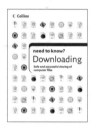 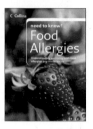 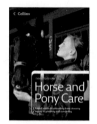

DJ Tips & Techniques — Dog and Puppy Care — Downloading — Food Allergies — Horse and Pony Care

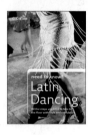 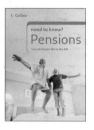 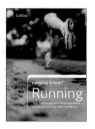 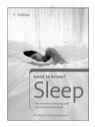 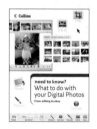

Latin Dancing — Pensions — Running — Sleep — What to do with your Digital Photos

Other titles in the series:

To order any of these titles, please telephone 0870 787 1732 quoting reference 263H. For further information about all Collins books, visit our website: www.collins.co.uk